50p

Psyche and Helix

Psyche and Helix

Psychological Aspects of Genetic Counseling

Essays by Seymour Kessler, Ph.D.

Edited by Robert G. Resta, M.S.

Division of Perinatal Medicine
Swedish Medical Center
Seattle, Washington

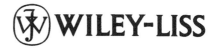

A JOHN WILEY & SONS, INC., PUBLICATION

NEW YORK • CHICHESTER • WEINHEIM • BRISBANE • SINGAPORE • TORONTO

Copyright © 2000 by Wiley-Liss, Inc. All rights reserved.

Published simultaneously in Canada.

For ordering and customer service, call 1-800-CALL-WILEY.

Library of Congress Cataloging-in-Publication Data:

Psyche and helix : psychological aspects of genetic counseling / edited by Robert G. Resta ; essays by Seymour Kessler.
    p. cm.
   Includes index.
   ISBN 0-471-35055-9 (alk. paper)
    1. Genetic counseling—Psychological aspects. I. Kessler, Seymour. II. Resta, Robert G.

  RB155.7 .P78 2000
  616'.042—dc21

                                                00-020717

Printed in the United States of America.
10 9 8 7 6 5 4 3 2 1

To Susan, Emily, and Lizzie.

—RR

To my grandchildren, who speak for the future.

—SK

Contents

Preface   *Robert G. Resta*   ix

1. **Analysis of a Transcript**   1

2. **Quantitative Analysis of a Transcript of a Genetic Counseling Session**   19

3. **Management of Guilt and Shame**   35

4. **Suffering and Countertransference**   63

5. **Preselection: A Family Coping Strategy in Huntington Disease**   68

6. **Advanced Counseling Techniques**   73

7. **More on Counseling Skills**   85

8. **Empathy and Decency**   99

9. **A Critical Review of the Literature Dealing with Education and Reproduction**   109

10. **Teaching and Counseling**   135

11. **Thoughts on Directiveness**   142

12. **Nondirectiveness Revisited**   150

13. **Notes and Reflections**   165

    Index   173

Preface

Genetic counseling has been defined in many ways since Sheldon Reed first coined the phrase more than 50 years ago (Resta, 1997). Depending upon the training and philosophical bent of the practitioner, genetic counseling has been viewed as an exercise in risk calculation, psychosocial assessment, education about medical and genetic information, a communication process, or a euphemism for eugenics. In some ways, all of these definitions are correct. After all, genetic counseling is defined by the practice of professionals who call themselves genetic counselors. Genetic counseling *is* what genetic counselors *do*.

So what should a genetic counselor *do* during a counseling session? Counselees almost always answer that question. Sometimes we can simply ask clients what they want from us (Michie et al., 1997). Often, though, we must rely on clinical skills and experience to elicit from patients what they want to gain from their time with us. Whatever agenda the counselor brings to the table, what matters most is what is important to counselees (Michie et al., 1998). If clients are not interested in discussing Bayesian risk calculation, population improvement, their innermost feelings, DNA mutations, or whatever a counselor *believes* is important to patients, then the session is for naught (Berkenstadt et al., 1999; Shankar et al., 1999). Everybody loses. Clients come away frustrated, their needs unmet (Freyer et al., 1999; McGowan, 1999). Counselors are left puzzled about why they cannot get through to counselees and become annoyed at the latter's inability to understand technical information despite the counselor's valiant efforts to explain it.

One way to help assure a rewarding counseling experience is to dispel the notion that clients who come for genetic counseling are primarily seeking education. This is not to say that clinical and educational issues are not important to them (Smith, 1998). Indeed, receiving a diagnosis and having the diagnosis and testing options explained are very important aspects of client satisfaction (Berkenstadt et al., 1999;

McCarthy Veach et al., 1999; Michie et al., 1997). But if education is the primary goal of genetic counseling, then a well-written book, Internet site, or a CD-ROM could better serve patients.

I argue that genetic counseling is more than an exercise in specialized education. At its core, genetic counseling is about helping people try to understand and cope with the effects of genetic disease on their lives and the lives of their families (Street and Soldan, 1998). Genetic counseling touches on the emotions and behaviors that define us as human—suffering, sacrifice, reproduction, self-image, family relationships, guilt, joy, anger, denial, love, and the struggle to comprehend the unpredictable world in which we live (Taswell and Sholtes, 1999). Indeed, genetic counseling is a *de facto* psychological process (Reif and Baitsch, 1985; Shiloh, 1996). A client's understanding of, and reaction to, any information we provide is shaped by a complex filter composed of the client's unique psychological makeup, emotional status, age, sex, culture, and developmental and personal experiences (Finucane, 1998; Lippman, 1999). As much as we might want to believe otherwise, counselees do not plan a perfectly logical course of reproductive or medical action based on a mathematical weighing of risks and advantages. People are not, in the words of songwriter Tom Waits, "bone machines."

Because genetic counseling can raise so many psychological issues, should genetic counselors be psychotherapists? No, at least they should not be psychotherapists *sensu strictu*. Most genetic counselors are neither trained as psychotherapists, nor do most genetic counseling patients suffer from psychopathology. Nevertheless, good counseling requires the counselor to have certain basic counseling skills:

- The ability to understand the psychological needs of others.
- The ability to understand the psychological meaning of clients' behaviors.
- The ability to communicate that understanding in ways that leave clients emotionally enriched, psychologically stronger, and more competent to deal with their own lives.

We also need to recognize that the very act of genetic counseling may result in a psychotherapeutic experience for the client. Learning about the cause of a child's mental retardation may help alleviate the guilt of a mother who had blamed her child's problems on a medication she took while she was pregnant, or some kind words from a counselor offered at the appropriate time during a session may help a patient come to terms with his or her disorder (Targum, 1981; Eunpu, 1997; Matloff, 1997; Resta, 1998; Tuttle, 1998; Biesecker and Marteau, 1999; Peters et al., 1999). But many patients who seek genetic counseling are not in need of the long-term specialized care of a psychotherapist, or should be referred to a psychotherapist when appropriate.

While genetic counselors need not be full-time psychotherapists, they do need to demonstrate basic counseling skills to achieve the goals of genetic counseling. A genetic counselor must be able to calculate risks, provide clear and accurate information about complex medical issues, and possess good administrative skills. But even the most complex risk calculation is a useless statistic if the counselor does not possess the ability to help the client put that risk in a meaningful and appropriate psychological context. What does it matter if a 35-year-old woman has "only" a 5% risk for developing ovarian cancer if the counselor does not understand that the woman has refrained from having children because she would not want her young children to watch her die from this disease at a young age, just like she watched her own mother die 20 years ago? A counselor might not understand a woman's ambivalence about undergoing amniocentesis unless the counselor knows that as a child the woman mercilessly teased the neighbor boy who was mentally retarded, and feels that she should be "punished" by making her first-born child have Down syndrome.

There are many excellent books and articles about clinical genetics and the calculation of recurrence risks. There are very few publications that provide practical and clinically meaningful ways to enhance the counseling skills of genetic counselors. Dr. Kessler's essays form the largest systematic approach to understanding and applying basic counseling skills to the practice of genetic counseling. Published over two decades in *American Journal of Medical Genetics* and *Journal of Genetic Counseling*, the essays retain their crispness and relevance to the daily practice of genetic counseling.

Many people contributed to the development of this book and the essays and we are most grateful to them, especially Dr. John Opitz, Dr. Charles Epstein, Pat Ward, Hilda Kessler, A.G. Jacopini, Dr. Alan Leveton, Colette Bean and Luna Han at John Wiley and Sons, Inc., Carol Prince, and Kluwer Academic/Human Sciences Press.

REFERENCES

Berkenstadt M, Shiloh S, Barkai G, Katznelson M B-M, Goldman B (1999) Perceived personal control (PPC): a new concept in measuring outcome of genetic counseling. Am J Med Genet 82:53–59.

Biesecker BB, Marteau TM (1999) The future of genetic counseling: an international perspective. Nat Genet 22:133–137.

Eunpu D (1997) Systematically-based psychotherapeutic techniques in genetic counseling. J Genet Counsel 6:1–20.

Finucane B (1998) Working with Women Who Have Mental Retardation. Elwyn, PA: Elwyn, Inc.

Freyer G, Dazord A, Schlumberger M, Conte-Devoix B, Ligneau B, Trillet-Lenoir V, Lenoir GM (1999) Psychosocial impact of genetic testing in familial medullary-thyroid carcinoma: a multicentric pilot-evaluation. Ann Oncol 10:87–95.

Lippman A (1999) Embodied knowledge and making sense of prenatal diagnosis. J Genet Counsel 8:225–274.

Matloff ET (1997) Generations lost: a cancer genetics case report. J Genet Counsel 6:169–186.

McCarthy Veach P, Truesdell SE, LeRoy BS, Bartels DM (1999) Client perceptions of the impact of genetic counseling. J Genet Counsel 8:191–216.

McGowan R (1999) Beyond the disorder: one parent's reflection on genetic counselling. J Med Ethics 25:195–199.

Michie S, Marteau TM, Bobrow M (1997) Genetic counselling: the psychological impact of meeting patients' expectations. J Med Genet 34:237–241.

Michie S, Weinman J, Marteau T (1998) Genetic counselors' judgments of patient concerns: concordance and consequences. J Genet Counsel 7:219–232.

Peters JA, Djurdjinovic L, Baker D (1999) The genetic self: The Human Genome Project, genetic counseling and family therapy. Fam Syst Health 17:5–25.

Reif M, Baitsch H (1985) Psychological issues in genetic counselling. Hum Genet 70:193–199.

Resta R (1997) Sheldon Reed and fifty years of genetic counseling. J Genet Counsel 6:375–378.

Resta R (1998) Carolyn's feet. Am J Med Genet 72:1–2.

Shankar A, Chapman P, Goodship J (1999) Genetic counseling: do we recognise and meet the consultands' agenda? J Med Genet 36:580–582.

Shiloh S (1996) Genetic counseling: a developing area of interest for psychologists. Prof Psychol Res Prac 27:475–486.

Smith ACM (1998) Patient education. In: Baker D, Schuette JL, Uhlmann WR (eds). *A Guide to Genetic Counseling*. New York: Wiley-Liss, pp 99–126.

Street E, Soldan J (1998) A conceptual framework for the psychosocial issues faced by families with genetic conditions. Fam Syst Health 16:217–232.

Targum S (1981) Psychotherapeutic considerations in genetic counseling. Am J Med Genet 8:281–289.

Taswell HF, Sholtes SK (1999) Predictive genetic testing: a story of one family. Fam Syst Health 17:111–121.

Tuttle LC (1998) Experiential family therapy: an innovative approach to the resolution of family conflict in genetic counseling. J Genet Counsel 7:167–186

1

Analysis of a Transcript[1]

INTRODUCTION

Although much has been written about the goals and outcome of genetic counseling, little is known about the actual content, structure, and dynamics of the counseling session itself (Fraser, 1974). Available information generally represents an idealized view of what genetic counseling might or should be; knowledge of what actually transpires is scanty or virtually nonexistent. Kelly (1977) has published a transcript of a postcounseling follow-up visit, and Kessler (1979a) has recently published partial transcripts of genetic counseling sessions. Several videotapes of genetic counseling sessions are known to the author but are not widely available; little encouragement is given to genetic counselors who wish to make audio- or videotapes of their work. Also present in the genetic counseling literature are several accounts of what counselors have reported to have said in response to requests for advice from genetic counselors (e.g., Fraser, 1977), These reports are difficult to evaluate since they are invariably presented out of context and some appear to paraphrase what was said rather than present a verbatim record.

The lack of information about what actually goes on in genetic counseling has impeded the identification of areas in which counseling practices might be made more effective, as well as those in which success has been achieved. Thus, it is difficult, if not impossible, to upgrade underlying concepts and improve practices where such are needed and, conversely, to take full pride in achievements when they occur. Also, since the content and process variables of the genetic counseling

[1]This essay first appeared as Kessler S (1981) Psychological aspects of genetic counseling: analysis of a transcript. *American Journal of Medical Genetics* 8:137–153. Reprinted with kind permission of the publisher, John Wiley and Sons.

session have not been delineated, outcome research has been limited. Thus, steps to increase our understanding of the content and process of the genetic counseling session need to be welcomed. To that end, a transcript of a genetic counseling session is presented here.

The session involves preamniocentesis counseling, currently a rather common situation in genetic counseling clinics. The performance of the counselor in this session is not held out as a model of what genetic counseling should be. On the contrary, the counseling is not exemplary of quality listening or response skills and of high levels of empathy. Many counseling errors will be apparent, and some of these will be noted. (The reader will probably recognize others not underscored.) The reader should consider that the purpose of presenting this transcript is not to evaluate the counselor, but to illustrate psychological issues. It should also be kept in mind that at the time of the actual counseling the counselor had not known that his work would be subjected to scrutiny or that the session would be evaluated for psychological issues. We are indebted to the counselor, who desires anonymity, for sharing his work with us.

The transcript has been edited to assure anonymity. Omitted portions are generally summarized so that the thread of the content is not lost. Each transaction is numbered on the left so that referral to specific points is facilitated in later discussion. The grammar is that of the original.

Following the transcript, the comments of two separate readers, Dr. Alan Leveton and myself, will be presented. In our separate evaluations, we will focus more on the process of the session, rather than on its content. Among other things, we will comment on the procedures used by the counselor, his style of counseling, the nature of his interaction with the counselees, the personality characteristics of the participants, defensive maneuvers, and some of the psychological issues raised in the session.

Process evaluation of verbatim transcripts is a standard procedure in the training of mental health professionals. Its educational value lies in the fact that it allows the trainees to gain distance from their work so that the less obvious features of the counseling landscape stand out in larger relief. It gives people an opportunity to observe the consequences of their interventions and of their own actions, defensive and otherwise, interacting with the clients. In addition, one has an opportunity to reflect on what one has said and to imagine and rehearse more effective ways of proceeding that may be useful in future sessions.

The transcript concerns a couple, a husband (H) and wife (W), in their early forties referred for routine preamniocentesis counseling because of W's age. The counselees are of average intelligence (counselor's estimate). H is a laborer; W is a housewife. Other pertinent information about the counselees will emerge in the course of the transcript. Prior to the outset of the session, the counselor (C), a male, has introduced himself to H and W in the waiting room and has obtained their consent to tape the session. Together they have proceeded to a nearby room in which three chairs are arranged in a triangular fashion. The first transaction occurs as the participants are seating themselves.

TRANSCRIPT

1. W: Are you the doctor who's going to do the test?

2. C: No, I'm one of the genetic counselors who are part of the genetic counseling clinic.

3. W: You don't do the test then?

4. C: I don't do the test—

5. W: [*interrupts*] What do you do, just tell us what the test is all about?

6. C: That's correct, I talk to you about what the test is all about. [*pause*] Perhaps that might be a good place to start. What was your understanding about why we're meeting today?

7. W: Well, Dr. A at Central City said that women over 35 years old usually have this test when [*unclear*], and they can test if and see if there's any. If it's retarded, I don't want to have it.

8a. C: Did he tell you about our meeting right now? We're not going to do the test now—

9a. W: [*interrupts*] No, they—

8b. C: Did you have any idea about why we're meeting today?

9b. W: —no, the Omega Medical Center called me and said that we're, me and my husband, are supposed to be here at 10 o'clock, and then we'd discuss it, and then I'd have to get another appointment to come back and have it done.

10. C: Right. Was this your understanding, Mr. G.?

11. H: Yeah, right.

12. W: I guess we're supposed to discuss this and see if we want it done, I don't know.

13. C: Okay, that's my understanding of why we're meeting. [*to H*] You were going to say something?

14. H: No, I was just going to say, it's never happened before, and it's kind of new to us, but with some of the methods done—

15. C: Uh, huh.

16. W: [*interrupts*] Has this been done much?

17. C: Yes, it's been done quite a bit.

18. W: How many years would you say?

19. C: Oh, we started doing this procedure I'd say over 10 years ago, but it's really in the last 5 years—

20. W: [*interrupts*] Then it's really not done experimentally.

21. C: This is not an experimental procedure. There are papers published on the safety of it. I'll discuss that with you, but I can just tell you right now that it's considered to be a very safe procedure both for the mother and the fetus.

[*pause*] Well what I would like to focus on, if I can for a moment, you say this is a surprise, and the thing that occurs to me is, you are how old Mrs. G?

22. W: 40.

23. C: And you Mr. G.?

24. H: 43.

25. C: 43. Okay. And do you have any children?

26. W: Two.

27. C: You have two children.

28. W: Adopted children.

29. C: In other words, you have no biological—

30. W: [*interrupts*] No, they're my children, but they're adopted.

31. C: Is this the only marriage for the two of you?

32. W: Yes.

33. [*C continues to focus on taking a family history. He asks several questions, among which the following exchange occurs:*]

34. C: To the best of your knowledge, are there any major diseases that run in the family on your side or on your side?

35. W: Cancer.

36. C: Cancer. What kind? Breast cancer?

37. W: Just cancer, I don't know what kind it is, just cancer, of the uterus. My mother got it, and she's still alive. All my uncles and grandmother and grandfather, they all died of it, on my father's side.

38. C: On your father's side.

39. W: But my mother got cancer, but she's okay now.

40. C: Do *you* have any concerns about that?

41. W: Oh, yeah, but I go to the doctor and get my Pap smear.

42. C: [*to H*] How about you?

43. H: My mother died of a heart attack, and I just had a brother in 1973 died of a massive heart attack. He was 43 years old.

44. C: Do you have any concerns about yourself? About heart attacks?

45. H: Yeah, I, it runs through my mind. I don't worry about it to the extent that—

46. W: [*interrupts*] If it happens—

47. H: —if I have one, hell, if it's going to happen it's going to happen. I usually try to get a physical once a year.

48. C: That's wise.

49. [*C asks several other health questions.*]

50. C: All right, let me tell you about the procedure. It's a procedure called amniocentesis. Essentially it's done. Let me find a picture of it [*opens pamphlet*].

51. W: With a needle.

52. C: That's right.

53. W: Do they take X-rays to see where the baby's at or they know?

54. C: Well, I'm going to talk about that. Then they introduce, they give some local anesthetic so that you won't feel the puncture. You'll probably feel some pressure, and they'll put the needle into this cavity where the fetus is [*points to picture*].

55. [*C addresses himself to the concerns that most people raise about the procedure, i.e., fetal damage and the possibility of spontaneous abortion. He describes the results of the National Institute of Child Health and Human Development study and ends by stating that there is no strong evidence that the procedure will induce a higher-than-average rate of miscarriage. He then says:*]

56. C: Now, I would like you stop me at any point if you have questions. Any time you really don't understand me, I'll be glad to go over it again.

57. W: Is this proven that they always know, I mean like if they do this and they found this mental problem, then they take the baby out? How do they—

58. C: [*interrupts*] Let's talk about why do they take the fluid out and what happens to that fluid after they take it out.

59. [*C continues by systematically describing the culture of amniotic fluid cells and the visualization of the chromosomes. He informs them that it will take from 3 to 4 weeks to obtain the laboratory results following the tap. He briefly describes the function of genes and chromosomes and the process of gametogenesis. He continues:*]

60. C: Sometimes it happens that the chromosomes don't divide correctly, so that instead of there being the normal number, there's either one less or one more. That's the thing that we're going to be looking for in our laboratory when we look at the chromosomes. Now one of the major conditions that we're going to look for is something called the Down syndrome. Have you ever seen a child like this? [*Shows picture.*] Mongoloid child?

61. W: Yes.

62. C: That's Down syndrome. That's what a child with Down syndrome looks like. And the cause of Down syndrome has been known to be due to the fact that there's an extra chromosome present in this chromosome group [*points*]. This is what the chromosomes are going to look like when they're all stained and everything. These are photographs of chromosomes, and you notice that some are big and some are small. When you take these chromosomes, and you arrange them in size place, you come out with a picture called a karyotype. Here's a picture of what they look like when they put them in size place. This is a chromosome constitution of a male fetus.

63. W: Uh, hum.

64. C: There's an X chromosome and a Y chromosome. Only boys have an X and Y. Now females have two X chromosomes.

65. W: So they will be able to say if it's a boy or a girl.

66. C: That's right. Now. For each chromosome, they come in pairs. You contribute one and you contribute one . . . Sometimes it happens there's an extra chromosome, and when that occurs you get Down syndrome. And that occurs in about 1 in 700—

67. W: [*interrupts*] How about after the age of 40?

68. C: Okay, let me show you that [*points to graph*]. It's been known for many decades now that the older the mother, the higher the chances for Down syndrome occurring. So under age 30 you see it's very low [*points to graph*]; this is the incidence of 1000 births. So here you see under 30 it's very low, it's less than 1 per 1000. Here's your age group now [*points*], and you see what happens here, 1% or a little bit higher than 1%. That means 99 chances out of 100, you're not going to have a baby with Down syndrome, but there's a 1% chance that you will.

69. W: Well, what else do they look for besides the mongol, mental retarded—

70. C: [*interrupts*] Okay, as you probably know, Down syndrome is associated with mental retardation. That's one of the major symptoms associated with Down syndrome.

71. W: Down syndrome, is that mongoloid?

72. C: Mongoloid, the proper name of it is Down syndrome.

73. W: But that's mainly what they look for then is this.

74. C: They'll look for that plus any other chromosomal disorder. There are other disorders, and when you put them all together, a woman your age has about a 2% chance of having a child with any chromosomal disorder.

75. W: Especially when it's the first one after 22 years of marriage.

76. C: Now you've been married 22 years, so this is sort of like a surprise party. How do you feel about this? Do you want this baby?

77. W: Yeah, I do.

78. C: How about you Mr. G.?

79. H: Yeah, it's as you mentioned it earlier, it's a shock. But when we first got married, we went to doctors two, three, four, five, eight years after we got married, and they said there's nothing wrong with either one of us, and just keep trying.

80. W: We really gave up on it.

81. H: Then about after the eighth year we were married, we decided to adopt.

82. C: Uh, huh.

83. H: We got a girl, and then a year and a half, two years later, we got a boy; we adopted a boy, through the Children's Home Society of Central City.

84. C: How have you been enjoying them?

85. H: Beautiful.

86. W: They're just, I couldn't love my own any more, I think.

87. C: How old are they now?

88. H: The girl's 14, the boy's 12. So, then here we learned just a couple months ago, she kind of felt this regular kind of pregnancy sickness. I guess you'd call it that.

89. W: I thought I had a tumor though, I didn't dream, but still the doctor—

90. H: She went to see her doctor, and he said you're pregnant. So it's a little shocking—

91. C: Yeah, I bet.

92. H: —but it's great. I feel it's great.

93. W: Actually, neither one of us had our hopes up too much until after we've had some testing done.

94. H: Before she had missed two or three months some times.

95. W: Earlier, actually never two months, just one. This time I missed a whole month of July, and I had a little one in August and that was the last one, but I guess I was pregnant when I had that period. Dr. A., she told me about his test that we're probably going to have now. There were some questions, I felt the doctor knew best and everything that's kind of the way we'd go.

96. H: I wasn't familiar with all this stuff you're talking about now. I do have a couple of questions, but maybe I'm getting ahead—

97. C: No, no, go right ahead.

98. H: What guarantee is there there's not going to be a mistake in the lab?

99. C: That's a fair question to ask. So far as we know, we haven't made mistakes. But the chances of it are extremely small . . . So far as I know, we've never told parents that the child was normal, and it turned out to be a mongoloid child or something like that. I cannot, of course, give you a guarantee of that—

100. H: I was just wondering.

101. C: It's highly unlikely that that could happen.

102. H: What, uh, is there another, uh, I suppose the test showed that it would be abnormal?

103. C: Good, good. As I told you, once the sample of amniotic fluid is removed it takes about four weeks till we get our results. When they finally get to look at the chromosomes, we're pretty confident that we can give you an answer as to whether there's a normal chromosomal constitution or whether there's an abnormal one. Now have you given any thought to what's going to be if we do have to call you and tell you that the child has an abnormal chromosomal constitution? Have you thought about what you would do?

104. W: Which means that the baby would be like that?

105. C: Possibly.

106. W: What do you mean possibly now?

107. C: Well it could be *that* chromosomal disorder, or it might be some other chromosomal disorder that might be a little bit less or might be a little bit more severe.

108. W: No, we really haven't talked about it.

109. H: Oh, this was more reason for my question earlier, if it was an abnormal fetus [*unclear*], and then is there any other test?

110. C: No, it's the only test that can be done.

111. H: And that would be up to us to either say let it go or else let's take it.

112. C: That's right, you haven't given any thought—

113. W: No, really, we haven't really talked about it.

114. H: [*simultaneously*] No we haven't talked—

115. C: Do you have any feelings about it? I mean what's the thoughts off the top of your head?

116. W: I think that if it's like that [*points to picture of Down syndrome child*], we should abort it. I mean I'm not a real young woman, and he's not, and I wouldn't want to have a baby. I don't know, because I've never really seen anyone like, like that, are they mental or what?

117. C: They're mentally retarded—

118. W: [*interrupts*] They never—

119. C: —most of the chromosome disorders lead to mental retardation.

120. W: So it's like they never grow up, huh?

121. C: That's about it . . . They require a lot of more care than a normal child. Sometimes they have a lot of other problems besides the mental retardation like heart problems, bowel problems, things like that. They need special schools if it's possible to send them to school at all.

122. W: Do most women have them aborted when they know they're like this?

123. C: A lot of people have. Some people have decided, they have strong feelings about abortion, and have decided not to go ahead with the abortion . . . How about you Mr. G.?

124. H: I think I don't believe in abortion in the sense of the word. When it comes to a situation like this, I feel that if there's substantial proof that it's going to be abnormal, then I think I would go along with the abortion. I've been involved with people at work who have this type of children over the past 15, 20 years. Some of them have the child in homes, other homes, or schools or special schooling. I think, probably the hardship of what I have been informed of hearing them talk, and you can see it is disheartening—

125. W: [*interrupts*] There's no cure for any of this?

126. C: No, No.

127. H: I don't believe that personally right now I wouldn't want to go through that sort of thing, but it came to be, I would do it. But if there was a possibility of not doing it, I would probably do that.

128. W: Well, we don't really have to give an answer right now.

129. C: No, I'm not even asking you for one. I think it's something that I had to raise with you and ask for you to think about. 'Cause there's always that

small, 98 chances out of 100 that there won't be any problem, but there's always that 2% chance that—

130. H: [*interrupts*] Let me ask you a question.

131. C: Sure.

132. H: Have you been involved yourself, personally, or just contact or you phoned people back and said there is an abnormal fetus, and they've left it to have a normal birth and then see what came and let it go?

133. C: Well, personally, I have been involved in that. Most people have elected not to continue the pregnancy. They've decided to give it up and try again—

134. W: [*interrupts*] It would take us another 22 years [*laughs*].

135. H: Yeah, no I. Uh.

136. C: —I do know of cases where they've decided not to have an abortion because they were Roman Catholics, and they felt it was against their religion to kill a baby, I mean those are their words. So, they had the baby born—

137. W: [*interrupts*] And it was like that?

138. C: When we tell you that your child has an abnormal chromosome constitution, we're more than 99% positive of that evaluation. I know it's a difficult predicament, especially, if I take it, you have some feelings about abortion.

139. [*Following this exchange, C suggests that H and W need to discuss this matter between themselves further. C attempts to summarize his understanding of where the discussion has brought them. During this summary, H states that he feels that if the baby is healthy, it should be born, but if it had a disorder, then they should proceed with abortion. The issue of ultrasound was then brought up and discussed, and the cost of the various procedures was provided. W notices a pamphlet on Down syndrome and says:*]

140. W: Can I have this?

141. C: Yeah, sure . . . Let me just read you the consent form, so you know what you're signing. I take it you've both decided that you'd like to go ahead with this procedure.

142. W: [*to H*] Unless you want to take that form home and study and read it. I'd bring it back in. Or would I have to call to make an appointment?

143. C: You can bring it back with you.

144. W: 'Cause I would like to get an appointment. [*to H*] Do you want to take this home and study it?

145. H: Well, no, I don't think there's any need to.

146. W: Okay, we'll sign it here.

147. H: [*to W*] Do you have a pen?

148. C: Do you have any doubts? Questions?

149. W: No. [*firmly*]

150. C: [*to H*] Like I can try to put myself in your place, it's sort of a big step.

151. W: No, that's all right, what is this? [*She points to consent forms.*]

152. C: Okay, let me read this to you. [*He reads the form, finally stating:*] This procedure does not rule out the possibility of congenital defects to the fetus due to other causes. That's a point that I did not go over with you. So let me go over that one now. All we can do with this procedure, we can't perform miracles, we cannot guarantee that this child is going to be born without a genetic defect, or that the child will not be born with mental retardation due to some genetic defect. The only thing we can look at is to see if the chromosomes are normal. That's the only thing we can do with this procedure. That's where medical science is today. We can't do a gunshot kind of thing and try to detect the many other genetic diseases that exist.

153. W: But mental retardation, you can?

154. C: Mental retardation, due to chromosome disorders—

155. W: You mean there could be mental retardation due to something else?

156. C: That's correct—

157. W: Oh.

158. C: Those we cannot detect. One of the major causes of mental retardation due to genetic reasons is chromosomal disorders, so at least *that* can be ruled out. The frequency of chromosomal disorders and the mental retardation due to chromosomal disorders increases as the mother gets older. That's why the procedure is recommended for women who are above 35 years of age. I want to go over that again because this doesn't, all it can do is tell us whether or not the child has a chromosomal disorder, and these are, those the limitations.

159. H: Who would be doing this, getting the fluid?

160. C: It would be Dr. B., who's done all of them or virtually all of them.

161. W: Do they do this very often.

162. C: Yes, twice a week.

163. W: Just to one woman? I mean like two women a week is all?

164. C: Oh, no, no, no, they have a series of them. We usually have, like right now there are two other couples being counseled for the same procedure, and at 11 o'clock, there will be two more couples counseled.

165. W: What do you mean canceled?

166. C: Counseled. Just like we're doing, talking, it's called counseling—

167. W: Oh, counseling. I thought—

168. C: [*interrupts*] My New Jersey accent. It's like Jimmy Carter campaigning down South says, "Elect somebody in the White House who doesn't have an accent." I've got a New Jersey accent really bad. [*Everybody laughs.*]

169. [*C continues to read the consent form to the counselees. He informs them that excess amniotic fluid could be used, with their permission, for experimental purposes.*]

170. C: Well, we're just about winding down. You would sign here. Do you want to give permission for the use of excess material?

171. W: [*to H*] Do you?
172. H: It doesn't really matter, yeah.
173. W: What do most people put?
174. C: They usually say yeah.
175. W: Yeah, I guess so, maybe it'll help somebody in the future.

C had two further contacts with the counselees following the session. He met with them for a few minutes two weeks later while they were waiting for the amniocentesis procedure to be done. Final contact was by phone one month later, at which time C informed H and W that the chromosomes were okay. W asked what sex the fetus was going to be and was told she could expect a baby girl.

COMMENTS

Dr. Kessler

From the onset of the session, W asserts leadership. She appears to know something about the amniocentesis procedure and is clear about not wanting a retarded child (7). C has difficulty relating to her and tries unsuccessfully to involve H (10, 13). C picks up from H's statement, "It never happened before . . ." (14) that this pregnancy may be unplanned. He introduces the word "surprise" (21) as if the counselees had previously used it and begins to deal with the meaning of the pregnancy, but just as suddenly, he switches to taking a family and health history. He asks a question and supplies the answer himself (36), incorrectly it turns out. W underscores her mother's present health status (37, 39) as if to reassure herself and, possibly, to mitigate the threat posed by her identification with her mother.

H is the same age now as his brother was when the latter died. It would not be unusual if he had high concerns about his personal health at this point. As he begins to talk about his concern (45), W interjects, and H adopts a more reassuring tone, through bravado (47). One wonders about the rules of family functioning here. This couple may have an implicit rule that says one partner is not allowed to distress the other and thus must express personal concerns in a disguised way.

C moves on to describe the amniocentesis procedure and begins to say that a needle is involved, but never quite says it (50); W finishes his sentence (51). She appears to be ahead of C in terms of pacing and, possibly, of what she wants to know about the procedure.

C invites questions (56), and W responds immediately, but C first interrupts and then postpones supplying an answer (58) to her question. The two of them are still not on the same wavelength and remain so until W provides an opening (75) to finish the business begun earlier in the session (21) regarding the feelings about the pregnancy. C's show of empathy and interest (76, 84, 87, 91) appears to facilitate H's involvement, and the overall tone of the session changes.

W asks whether most women abort a Down fetus (122), and C tries to remain neutral by not supplying normative data (123). H appears to be relatively more reluctant than W with respect to abortion (124) and tries to find ways to avoid abortion, if at all possible.

C begins to read a consent form and appears to be pushing for closure (141). Toward the end of the session, an amusing exchange occurs (168) in which C shows a different side of himself. He is no longer the expert; he is a fallible human being just like the counselees.

In many respects, the genetic counseling session presented above is a rather ordinary one. No major surprises emerged, and no strong emotions were expressed. It lacks the drama and intensity of counseling sessions in which, for example, parents are informed of a serious diagnosis in their child or those in which anger or despair are expressed. In many respects, it is not atypical of many genetic counseling sessions.

The initial part of the session is conspicuous for the absence of a "warm-up" period, in which, through chitchat and conversational transactions, the participants become acquainted with each other, implicitly establish rules by which the session will proceed, and begin the definition of mutual role expectations (Kessler, 1979b). These transactions tend to reduce the generally high levels of anxiety attending the establishment of new social situations, particularly those of the client–professional relationship in health settings. W's opening series of terse questions (1, 3, 5) reflected the high level of anxiety she probably was experiencing. To manage and reduce this anxiety, her stylistic approach seemed to involve an active search for information and structure (Kessler, 1979c). Superficially, under such conditions, she appeared to be controlling and feisty, and C responded to her as if he experienced her behavior as involving a struggle for control. C appeared to have difficulty asserting leadership in the face of W's directiveness and courted H as an ally (10, 13, 97, 138). H's reserve, probably his way of handling anxiety, appeared to be more acceptable and less anxiety-provoking to C than W's behavior. C's major way of handling his initial anxiety was through attempts to contain the area of focus (21, 50, 54) and via postponements, that is, promising to emphasize the power aspects of the professional role and, because of their defensive nature, did not allow C to deal effectively with the feelings underlying the counselees' verbalizations.

In general, C had considerable difficulty dealing with affective material, at times ignoring it when obvious (7) or else evading direct involvement (21, 76, 115) with it. This difficulty led C to adopt an overall content-oriented approach (Kessler, 1979d), in which the major focus was on the presentation of information and factual material. He showed a relatively low level of empathy (Carkhuff and Berenson, 1967), particularly toward W. In contrast, he appeared to be supportive of H, rewarding the latter's questions with statements of approbation (99, 103), and attempting more direct empathic contact with him (138, 150).

Transaction 75 appeared to be a major pivotal point in the session. On a process level, the flow of the session had been interrupted by C's earlier deflection toward obtaining family history (21) just at the point when the "surprise" aspect of the pregnancy emerged. Later (75), W reminded C that the pregnancy was an unusually important event in their lives. It is at this point that C needed to choose between a response to the superficial content of W's statement or to its underlying metamessage (Satir, 1964; Kessler, 1979c). The content suggested that W believed, mistakenly, that her risk for an abnormal child was a function of or exacerbated by the fact that she was primigravida, whereas the metamessage emphasized that this pregnancy had important meanings for her. The impulse of many genetic counselors might be to focus on the counselee's mistaken belief and attempt to supply corrective factual information. This tactic would probably have been experienced as a lack of empathy, which might then have had further deteriorating consequences for the counselor–counselee relationship (Carkhuff and Berenson, 1967). The fact that at this point C acknowledged the special nature of the pregnancy for the counselees and inquired about their feelings regarding it conveyed to the counselees, for the first time, that he understood them. This intervention had several important consequences. The overall tone of the session changed. The counselees, particularly H, became more verbal and freer in their expression of feelings. There was a movement away from the staccato question–answer format to a more expansive, richer flow of verbalizations. Overall, there was less defensiveness and greater openness. The power struggle aspects of the session and the tensions and discomforts created by or associated with such controlling maneuvers diminished in intensity.

The two counselees appeared to have different personal agendas. W was relatively clear about wanting the amniocentesis test (7, 144) and about the possibility of an abortion (7, 116) if necessary. W appeared to be more conflicted about these issues: the safety of the procedures to herself and the fetus (16, 18, 20, 53, 159, 161, 163) and the possibility of having a mentally retarded child (57, 67, 69, 104, 116, 120, 153, 155). H, on the other hand, appeared to be more concerned about the issue of abortion and the possibility of aborting a normal fetus by mistake (98, 102, 109, 124, 127, 132), a situation that apparently would have violated his ethical standards (124). These differences in concerns between husbands and wives may be a widespread phenomenon among couples seeking, or referred for, amniocentesis (D. Beeson, personal communication).

Although no detailed content analysis was carried out, the material provided by C appeared to be adequate. With one surprising exception, the facts seemed ordered, moving from simpler to more complex concepts. Why C did not mention the limits of the disorders that could be detected via amniocentesis (152) earlier in the session is puzzling. On the whole, the level of vocabulary C used appeared appropriate.

Dr. Leveton

In reviewing this interview, I want to point out the disadvantages of using a history-taking style of interview, the questionable use of threatening information to obtain consent for procedures, and the missed opportunity for understanding the deeper issues crucial to the family. I also want to indicate some areas of general concern to the genetic counselor as a member of the clinical team.

C identifies himself as part of the clinic (2) and states that he is going to talk with H and W about the "test" (6). He presents himself as an expert and as a representative of a medical team. Much of C's interaction with the family follows the model of medical history-taking. He pursues facts and teaches the family to be passive while he asks the questions. In the same mode, he gives information and answers their questions, for the most part, factually and with little or no opportunity to find out the implication of their questions or impact of his information. As a consequence of C's history-taking style, H and W are rather limited to answering his questions and asking theirs (21). When he discovers a history of cancer and heart disease, he lets the matter drop. H has lost a brother at age 43 through a heart attack. W interrupts (46), and H takes a devil-may-care stance, and C allows the theme to close on the information that H gets a yearly physical. There are important unexplored clues here that are relevant to the matter at hand. Is it characteristic for W to protect her husband by interrupting or distracting? Are they concerned about the available energy and longevity needed for rearing even a normal newborn?

C shifts his agenda (50) to the "test" and its meaning. He knows many facts and gives them to the parents. He is so far within the medical education model that he talks to them of genes, chromosomes, gametogenesis, and karyotypes. He has no way to gauge if the parents understand his technical terms or to what use they put his information. Although he makes a token offer to "stop me if you have questions" (56), when the wife does (57), he interrupts (58) and continues with his explanations.

When experts explain to nonexperts, it is essential that they at least ask the non-expert to "say back to me in your own words what I have been trying to explain to you so that I can tell if I have been clear." Polite patients often try to save us embarrassment by nodding and simulating agreement when we have flooded them with jargon.

C has come prepared with graphs, photos, pamphlets about Down syndrome and the risk of chromosomal disorder occurring in this pregnancy. He is following his agenda to obtain consent for amniocentesis. There is no preparation for this visual confrontation. He neither asks what they may already know, nor asks if they are interested in seeing this picture. Nor does the counselor leave room for exploring any reaction they might have. This flood of facts, jargon, and photography takes up a major part of the interview. He is so immersed in statistics and diagnosis there is no room for H and W to comment on the unexpected materialization of a picture of a frightening possibility.

It would be far more useful to begin with letting the couple inform us about their response to the fact of pregnancy after 22 years of marriage and two adoptions. It would help to learn not only what they talk about between themselves and other family members, who often play a major role in giving or undermining support, but how they talk to one another.

Somewhere in this interview, we want the genetic counselor to find out, for example, if H and W feel free to raise questions, respect differences of opinion between themselves, and resolve conflicts. This would help make an assessment of how they will cope with whatever the pregnancy might bring and would help to identify future needs.

In his rather relentless evocation of the negative, C confronts them with the possibility of a phone call informing them that W is carrying an abnormal child (103). So far, in a perfunctory way, he has asked once, "Do you want this baby?" (76). It is unclear how they are adapting to the pregnancy. He now precipitates a premature discussion of abortion. The mental picture the wife has of the photo she has been shown makes her ask, "Which means the baby would be like that?" (137).

There is an interviewing dilemma here. The counselor should not be a Pollyanna who merely reassures that all will be for the best, nor should he, as he does here, rush ahead of the couple's capacity to assimilate new information. Opening a discussion of abortion sets up a decision-making about an issue that need not yet be confronted. Naturally, this is a highly charged area of discussion.

C gives facts and more facts; about associated defects, special schools (121), what other families might do (123). His preoccupation with the negative outcome is further reflected in his gratuitous information about Roman Catholics who feel it is "against their religion to kill a baby, . . . So they had the baby born—" [136]. The unexplored impact of the photo can be inferred by the wife's immediate response, "[interrupts] and it was like that?" [137].

W wants to take a pamphlet on Down syndrome; the counselor merely says "Yeah, sure" [141]. No one knows what she intends to do with it.

The last part of the interview has C pursuing his major objective, obtaining their signature on the consent form for amniocentesis. How remote his agenda is from what theirs may be can be seen in his last transaction with them. He wants use of the excess amniotic fluid for experimental purposes. Whose needs are being served here? An ending that would be client-centered would have the counselor identifying himself as a person available for further discussion, available if conflict or trouble develops, and available through the process of this pregnancy and its outcome.

This interview demonstrates some of the pitfalls that lie in wait for the genetic counselor who is unclear about what is needed for counseling families that find themselves facing difficult dilemmas related to highly worrisome prospects in bearing children. This counselor's main goal is to explain a procedure (amniocentesis) and obtain consent to perform it. It is likely he will miss important larger issues facing the family. These parents are in a situation of hope, anxiety, and possibly disappointment, loss, and tragedy. The counselor neither explores the emotional situation of the family nor discovers their patterns of interaction; nor does he offer informed emotional support.

The special function of the genetic counselor should be to help family members achieve understanding of their experience in difficult circumstances. He should be in a position to know about their patterns of communication and miscommunication, about fears and guilt, and about their potential for mutual support. In family therapy terms, it means understanding *process* (how people relate) rather than focusing on *content* (the facts given and taken). History-taking and factual explanation can probably be done equally well by other members of the genetic services team. The counselor has as his province helping people navigate the dilemmas and ambiguities of pregnancy clouded by special circumstances.

The background and interests of genetic counselors are generally heavily scientific and medical. They are often not prepared to deal with the deep emotions necessarily associated with the kind of caseload they encounter. They are most comfortable with facts and least comfortable with feelings. They want to actively do things and have trouble letting interviews develop in a way that might reveal the family situation. They frequently want to distract people away from tears and anger and hope to help people avoid pain through factual knowledge. The clientele of genetic counseling clinics are often heavily burdened with tears and anger.

Because genetic counselors often deal with families that have experienced loss and are confronted with great ambiguity and possible tragedy, it is important that they be trained to interview families and remain competent and comfortable in the presence of deep emotional feelings and to understand the special needs in this situation. They need to understand how events can go well or poorly as families encounter institutional settings as well as the particular dynamics of their genetic counseling team. Counselors, of necessity, will need to confront deep philosophic issues relating to the quality of life, love, and sacrifice in families, death, and loss. All this encompasses what is comprehensive about comprehensive care; so easy to advocate and so difficult to deliver.

DISCUSSION

In our separate comments, Dr. Leveton and I are substantially in agreement on many of the issues raised by this counseling session, particularly those concerning process. There is agreement on C's general inability to deal effectively with affective material and his basic use of a counseling style that emphasizes content (or, as Dr. Leveton puts it, medical history-taking) at the expense of process issues. The issues on which we do not seem to agree are relatively minor ones. For example, Dr. Leveton's reading of the transcript leads him to suggest that C may have been providing new information at a pace that outstripped the couple's capacity to assimilate it. My reading leads me to an opposite conclusion; that is, that C has underestimated the counselee's capacity in this regard, at least at certain points of the session.

The genetic counselor's style of counseling deserves greater discussion because it touches on the broader interrelated issues of counselor directiveness and neutrality and his role as an educator. The traditional model of genetic counseling has emphasized the provision of information and has promoted a counseling stance in which the counselor performed as a neutral educator. This approach was a transposition of the ambiance and methods of the classroom to the counseling situation.

In the session above, C appears to play a nondirective, neutral educator role. He provides facts and information. When asked to provide advice or normative data (122, 132), he attempts to tread a somewhat middle course, refraining from giving direct advice. Is this being nondirective? Yes, but only if we narrowly define "nondirective" as meaning that he has not told the counselees what to do in the area of future reproduction. However, in a broader sense, C has been most directive in that his interventions have been aimed (consciously or otherwise) at influencing the counselees' behavior so that they will agree to have the amniocentesis procedure. For example, take C's use of pictures of a Down syndrome child, photographs of chromosomes, and graphs showing the relationship between risks and advancing maternal age. This practice is based on standard pedagogic techniques and seems consistent with the neutral educator model of genetic counseling. Furthermore, it is a practice endorsed by many genetic counselors (e.g., Fuhrmann and Vogel, 1969; Reynolds et al., 1974; Davis, 1979) as a means of imparting information, facilitating learning, and clarifying complex issues. It probably is a widely used strategy in genetic counseling. However, such practices may also serve other, perhaps unintended ends by focusing the counselees' attentions on the likelihood of having a defective child rather than a normal child and thus cognitively magnifying their risk for an affected child. This may be a means of arousing their anxieties, fears, and aversions regarding birth defects and of increasing their motivation (or triggering existing motivations) to take appropriate actions to avoid such a problem. Thus, out of context, as an isolated episode, C's behavior might easily be assessed as an attempt at educating the counselees. In context with the remainder of the session, his behavior appears more to be an exercise in persuasion. These differing perspectives emerge large because of the differences provided by a content versus a process focus.

Antley (1979), Hsia (1979), and others have been critical of the myth of the unbiased, nondirective counselor in genetic counseling. The information provided in genetic counseling is not emotionally neutral (Kessler, 1979d), and how such information is provided has cognitive and affective consequences for the counselees (Pearn, 1973). Hsia (1979) has suggested that merely raising the issue of prenatal diagnosis implies an endorsement not only of the procedure, but of abortion of an affected fetus as well. These considerations suggest that greater attention needs to be given to the implied messages or metamessages (Kessler, 1979c) genetic counselors transmit to counselees, for these, rather than the content of genetic counseling, may exert the major influence on later decision-making.

Elsewhere (Kessler, 1979b), it has been suggested that genetic counseling, like all other forms of personal counseling, can be understood as an attempt to influence behavior. In genetic counseling, an influence is being exerted on counselees' attitudes, beliefs, or its sequelae. Providing factual information may help counselees reorganize their thinking about genetic disease, which may then lead to actions not previously contemplated. Dealing with counselees' feelings of guilt, among others, is a direct effort to alter their cognitive and affective functioning. Whether we want it to be this way or not, genetic counselors are agents of behavior change (Kessler, 1979b, 1979e).

Heretofore, discussions of the issues of directiveness and counselor neutrality in the genetic counseling literature have generally been carried out in a limited and somewhat abstract way. Discussions of directiveness have frequently focused on the one issue of providing advice on reproduction. Discussions of neutrality have generally proceeded without a connection to specific procedures and interventions. These issues now need to be re-evaluated in terms of specific practices and procedures of genetic counseling. To do so, we need more information about what actually goes on in the genetic counseling session. Without such information, discussions of these issues will continue to remain in the abstract sphere.

CONCLUSION

Examination of a transcript of a genetic counseling session has revealed many of the limitations of a content-oriented style of counseling. A focus on affective material has been minimized. Thus, the issues bearing on the counselees' health behavior, their feelings about the current pregnancy, their decision regarding amniocentesis, and their potential decision about future abortion have all been superficially explored. Viewed from a process level, the counselor's counseling strategies appear to have been directed toward persuading the counselees to have the amniocentesis procedure. The one intervention displaying the counselor's awareness of the counselees' feelings appeared to have a positive impact on the remainder of the session in terms of improving the counselor–counselee relationship.

There is little reason to believe this session is atypical of genetic counseling sessions carried out by other counselors under similar circumstances. Further study of the content and process of genetic counseling is needed to identify areas where greater effectiveness might be achieved.

ACKNOWLEDGMENT

At the time this manuscript was written, Dr. Alan Leveton was Assistant Clinical Professor of Psychiatry and Pediatrics at University of California, San Francisco Medical Center and Director of the Family Therapy Center of San Francisco. I would like to thank Dr. Leveton for reading this manuscript and providing his comments and perspectives.

REFERENCES

Antley RM (1979) The genetic counselor as a facilitator of the counselee's decision process. Birth Defects: Original Article Series 15(15C):137–168.

Carkhuff RR, Berenson BG (1967) Beyond Counseling and Psychotherapy. New York: Holt, Rinehart and Winston.

Davis JG (1979) A counselor's viewpoint. Birth Defects: Original Article Series 15:113–122.

Fraser FC (1974) Genetic counseling. Am J Hum Genet 26:636–659.

Fraser FC (1977) Degrees of directiveness. In: Lubs HA, de la Cruz F (eds). Genetic Counseling. New York: Raven Press.

Fuhrmann W, Vogel F (1969) Genetic Counseling. New York: Springer-Verlag.

Hsia YE (1979) The genetic counselor as information giver. Birth Defects: Original Article Series 15(2):169–186.

Kelly PT (1977) Dealing with Dilemma. New York: Springer-Verlag.

Kessler S (1979a) The genetic counseling session. In: Kessler S (ed). Genetic Counseling: Psychological Dimensions. New York: Academic Press, pp 65–105.

Kessler S (1979b) The counselor–counselee relationship. In: Kessler S (ed). Genetic Counseling: Psychological Dimensions. New York: Academic Press, pp 53–63.

Kessler S (1979c) The process of communication, decision-making and coping in genetic counseling. In: Kessler S (ed). Genetic Counseling: Psychological Dimensions. New York: Academic Press, pp 35–51.

Kessler S (1979d) The psychological foundations of genetic counseling. In: Kessler S (ed). Genetic Counseling: Psychological Dimensions. New York: Academic Press, pp 17–33.

Kessler S (1979e) The genetic counselor as psychotherapist. Birth Defects 15(2):187–200.

Pearn JH (1973) Patients' subjective interpretation of risks offered in genetic counseling. J Med Genet 10:129–134.

Reynolds BD, Puck MH, Robinson A (1974) Genetic counseling: an appraisal. Clin Genet 5:177–187.

Satir V (1964) Conjoint Family Therapy. Palo Alto, CA: Science and Behavior Books.

2

Quantitative Analysis of a Transcript of a Genetic Counseling Session[1]

INTRODUCTION

Two major research approaches have been adopted in evaluating the effectiveness of counseling (or psychotherapy), study of outcome, and study of process (Korchin, 1976). Outcome research consists of an evaluation of the consequences of the counseling (or psychotherapy), whereas process research places the focus on what happened in the session itself. Obviously, it would be worthwhile to combine the two strategies by evaluating process variables and relating them to later outcome measures.

The effectiveness of genetic counseling has been virtually entirely evaluated by means of outcome studies (Shaw, 1977; Childs, 1978). These can be divided into three groups: (1) studies of reproductive attitudes and/or behavior, (2) studies of information recall, and (3) studies of affective changes. Generally, in individual studies, more than one facet of outcome has been examined.

The studies of reproductive attitudes and behavior have been equivocal in demonstrating changes as a result of genetic counseling (Childs, 1978). Some investigators have suggested that genetic counseling was effective in influencing family planning attitudes and activities (Carter et al., 1971; Emery et al., 1972; Reynolds et al., 1974; Lubs, 1979), whereas others have found little, if any, influence (Hsia, 1977; Black, 1979).

Results of studies of information recall are difficult to interpret. Some investigators suggest high levels of recall (e.g., Emery et al., 1972) following genetic counseling, but others do not (Sibinga and Freedman, 1971; Leonard et al., 1972). In some studies, no baseline data are given, and thus the extent of later recall cannot be attributed to the

[1]This essay first appeared as Kessler S, Jacopini AG (1982) Psychological aspects of genetic counseling. II. Quantitative analysis of a transcript of a genetic counseling session. *American Journal of Medical Genetics* 12:421–435. Reprinted with kind permission of the publisher, John Wiley and Sons.

genetic counseling. Recent data (Sorenson et al., 1980) suggest that only modest gains are obtained in postcounseling recall of diagnostic information and recurrence risks.

Studies of affective changes have shown that under some conditions genetic counseling may be effective in lowering anxiety (Antley and Hartlage, 1976), depression, and skepticism (Rowley et al., 1979) and in improving alertness (Rowley et al., 1979) as well as the person's overall self-concept (Antley et al., 1973; Antley and Hartlage, 1976; Corgan, 1979). Whether such changes are sustained and for how long are unknown, and it is unclear what specifically in the session might have led to such changes.

Many of the problems inherent in outcome studies of genetic counseling are due to a surprising paucity of information about what actually occurs within the counseling session itself. Without such information as to how the counseling was provided, the content of the session, what issues were emphasized, and what impact the professional had on the counselees, outcome measures will be difficult to assess. The need for process research on genetic counseling is long overdue, and, to our knowledge, the present investigations represent the first attempts at achieving some understanding of the process, content, and dynamics of genetic counseling.

The purposes of the present analysis were (1) to demonstrate the feasibility of applying quantitative methods to genetic counseling interactions, (2) to develop and apply operational measures of qualitative concepts (e.g., directiveness, content-orientation, etc.), and (3) to test hypotheses emerging from the previous qualitative analysis. Specifically, we wanted to test the following hypotheses:

Hypothesis 1. Counselor's (C) counseling style was content-oriented (Kessler, 1979a). By content-orientation we mean that the focus was overwhelmingly on the provision of medical information and genetic facts rather than on an attempt to explore personal meanings, attitudes, feelings, and dynamic issues.

Hypothesis 2. C's behavior toward the two counselees was significantly different; he showed a high level of "negativity" toward the wife (W) and was supportive of the husband (H).

Hypothesis 3. Transaction 76 marked a turning point in the session in which the quality of interactions prior to that transaction was different from those subsequent to it.

Hypothesis 4. The counseling style displayed by C was directive in that he was attempting to influence the counselees to have the amniocentesis procedure. In this regard, we are not attempting to express approval or disapproval of C's counseling style or behavior.

MATERIALS AND METHODS

The transcript of a genetic counseling session published by Kessler (1981) was the subject of the present analysis. The scoring system was developed by Bales (1950) to study small group interactions. This system involves three scoring procedures: *unitization,* in which various transactions are subdivided into scorable units; *categoriza-*

tion, in which each unit is assigned a category score (to be described below), and *attribution*, in which each unit is assigned a score designating the initiator and intended recipient(s) of the message inherent in the unit.

To score the transcript, the interactions between the participants were first divided into units. Unitization required the identification of the smallest discriminable segment of meaningful interaction to which a category score could be assigned. Sometimes the unit consisted of a single word, and at other times it consisted of part of, or a whole, sentence.

Each unit was assigned a category score (categorization) as follows:

1. Interactions showing solidarity with the other, raising the other's status, giving help or reward.
2. Interactions showing tension release, jokes, laughter, or satisfaction.
3. Interactions showing agreement, passive acceptance, understanding, concurrence, or compliance.
4. Interactions in which a suggestion or direction is given and autonomy for the other is implied.
5. Interactions in which an opinion, evaluation, or analysis is given or a feeling or wish is expressed.
6. Interactions in which orientation or information is provided or in which clarification or confirmation is given.
7. Interactions in which one asks for orientation, information, repetition, or confirmation.
8. Interactions in which one asks for an opinion, evaluation, analysis, or an expression of feeling.
9. Interactions in which one asks for a suggestion, direction, or possible action.
10. Interactions in which disagreement or passive rejection is shown or in which there is formality or a withholding of resources.
11. Interactions showing the presence of tension or in which one asks for help or permission or withdraws from the "interactive field."
12. Interactions in which one shows antagonism, defensiveness, or aggressiveness, or in which the other's status is deflated.

Each unit was assigned an attribution score designating the originator and intended recipient(s) of the message inherent in the unit. In all, nine attribution scores were possible:

- C–H, C–W, C–O, indicating a unit originating from the Counselor (C) directed, respectively, toward the Husband (H), the Wife (W), or both counselees (O);
- H–C, H–W, H–O, indicating, respectively, a unit originating from H and intended for C, W, or both C and W;
- W–C, W–H, W–O, indicating that the unit originated from W and directed, respectively, toward C, H, or both.

For a period of several weeks prior to scoring the transcript, the authors underwent an intensive training in the use of the Bales system. Another published transcript was used in this period, and, independently, the transcript was scored a section at a time. We met virtually every day to compare our respective scores, to discuss the points on which we disagreed, and to arrive at a consensus score for each unit. When it became apparent that we were in strong agreement on our scoring of the transcript, we decided to turn our attention to the present transcript. We continued to meet daily to compare our independent scores and to discuss and arrive at a consensus decision when differences occurred. We had a 79% rate of agreement on the scoring of units, an 84% rate of agreement on assigning category scores for individual units, and an 89% rate of agreement on assigning an attribution score.

In determining statistical significance, the data were arranged so as to use contingency or exact probability tables (Siegel, 1956).

RESULTS

Table 2.1 shows the frequency of scored categories for the individual participants in the session. Of the total number of units, C contributed 53.5%; W, 30.2%; and H, 16.3%.

If the units of H and W are combined, they comprise 46.5% of the total, nearly equal to the number scored for C. However, it should be noted that some material, which probably would have received scores in category 6, has been omitted in the published transcript (e.g., see transactions 33, 55, and 59). Thus, it is certain that the number of units attributed to C in the present analysis is an underestimate, particularly in the aforementioned category.

The most frequent categories, across participants, were, in order, 6, 5, and 7. Category 6 comprised 52.2% of all units; category 5, 13.8%, category 7, 10.4%; and the remaining categories comprised 23.6%.

The category scores were combined into four groups: A (categories 1, 2, 3), B (categories 4, 5, 6), C (categories 7, 8, 9) and D (categories 10, 11, 12), representing positive reactions, answers to questions, questions, and negative reactions respectively, and tested by means of a 2 × 4 contingency table. The scores of the counselor were significantly different ($\chi^2 = 24.9$, $P < .0001$) from those of the combined scores of H and W. C gave an almost threefold greater number of positive reactions and one-third less negative reactions than the counselees.

Table 2.1. Number of Units in Each Category for Participants in a Genetic Counseling Session

Participant	1	2	3	4	5	6	7	8	9	10	11	12	Total
C	18	2	10	18	25	165	16	19	0	1	3	6	283
H	0	1	3	0	21	47	7	1	0	0	6	1	87
W	0	4	3	0	27	64	32	2	3	3	6	15	159
Total	18	7	16	18	73	276	55	22	3	4	15	22	529

C = counselor, H = husband, W = wife.

Table 2.2. Attribution Characteristics of Scored Units

	Categories												
	1	2	3	4	5	6	7	8	9	10	11	12	Total
C–W	6	0	5	8	10	68	5	1	0	1	2	5	111
C–H	10	0	4	1	4	16	2	9	0	0	0	0	46
C–O	2	2	1	9	11	81	9	9	0	0	1	1	126
H–C	0	1	2	0	19	43	6	1	0	0	5	1	78
H–W	0	0	1	0	1	4	1	0	0	0	0	0	7
H–O	0	0	0	0	1	0	0	0	0	0	1	0	2
W–C	0	1	1	0	24	63	31	1	2	1	3	12	139
W–H	0	0	1	0	0	1	1	1	1	2	0	3	10
W–O	0	3	1	0	3	0	0	0	0	0	3	0	10
Total	18	7	16	18	73	276	55	22	3	4	15	22	529

C = counselor, H = husband, W = wife, O = both husband and wife.

Among the counselees, the total number of category scores for W was almost double that of H, and the distribution of scores in groups A, B, C, and D was significantly different ($\chi^2 = 12.12$; $P < .0001$) with the greatest difference occurring in the categories comprising groups C and D, where W showed more than a fourfold greater number of units in group C and a more than threefold greater number of units in group D than H did.

Table 2.2 shows the units arranged according to their attribution characteristics. W directed the overwhelming majority (87.5%) of her verbalization toward C. Similarly, H directed 90% of his verbalization toward C. The latter distributed his verbalizations as follows: 39.2% exclusively toward W, 16.3% exclusively toward H, and 44.5% toward both counselees.

C's direct interactions with H differed from those with W. There were more than a twofold greater number of direct interactions with W than with H. Nearly one-quarter of his direct interactions with H consisted of requests for information and opinions (categories 7, 8, and 9), whereas only 5.4% of C's interactions with W were such requests. Over 45% of C's direct interactions with H consisted of the provision of suggestions, opinions, and information (categories 4, 5, and 6), whereas 77.5% of his interactions with W were units in these categories. Of C's direct interactions with H, 21.7% were units of reward (category 1), whereas only 5.4% of his interactions with W showed such rewards.

In the interactions directed simultaneously to both counselees, most of C's units (80.2%) were in categories 4, 5, and 6.

Category Analysis

Pairs of categories in the Bales system of scoring might be conceived as attempts at solutions of functional problems encountered in interactional systems. Of particular interest are the pairs comprising categories 7 and 6, 8 and 5, and 9 and 4. Categories 7, 8, and 9 might be thought of as signals of difficulties, lacks, or needs to which categories 6, 5, and 4, respectively, are relevant attempts at repair and/or response. These sequences may be especially prominent in genetic counseling sessions and, because they bear on the hypotheses being examined here, warrant further attention.

Two methods were used to carry out a category analysis; the 7-6 sequence will be used for illustration purposes, with similar reasoning applying to 8-5 and 9-4 sequences. In method 1, the attribution characteristics of units were ignored and one scored the presence of unit of category 6 immediately following a unit of category 7. In method 2, one considered that units are frequently part of a larger transaction. For example, a question in category 7 might be followed immediately by explanatory information on the part of the originator of the question or, sometimes, another question. Thus, some questions may be embedded within the body of a transaction rather than appearing at the terminal portion of it. Similarly, answers to questions may also be embedded within a transaction surrounded by information and explanatory material rather than at the initial portion of a transaction. To account for this, the transcript was examined to determine the number of instances in which questions scored in category 7 were followed by a *transaction* (Kessler, 1981) in which at least one unit scored in category 6 occurred. Entire transactions between the originator and receiver of messages were scanned, and if at least one unit scored as 7 occurred in the transaction, the following transaction of the receiver was scored for the presence or absence of a unit in category 6. Only replies that were redirected to the sender were scored as being present.

Analysis of 7-6 sequences: Overall, there were 55 units scored in category 7 and 276 units scored in category 6. To apply method 1, five questions that had a rhetorical tone or otherwise did not call or expect an answer were omitted from the analysis. Thus, out of a total possible score of 50 (instances of units in category 7), only 31 (62%) were found to be followed by a unit in category 6.

Using method 2, it was found that 37 out of 42 transactions with at least one unit in category 7 (88.1%) were followed by a transaction in which at least one unit of category 6 occurred.

Analysis of 8-5 sequences: In all, there were 22 units scored in category 8 and 73 scored in category 5. Of the units in category 8, 19 occurred in transactions that allowed for response. Using method 1, as above, only two instances (10.5%) were found where a unit in category 8 was followed by one in category 5 (40.0%) out of 15 possible instances.

Analysis of 9-4 sequences: In all, there were three instances of units scored in category 9, and 18 in category 4. Of the three possibilities, only one unit in category 4 followed a transaction in which a unit in category 9 occurred (33.3%).

In summary, the analysis of 9-4, 8-5, and 7-6 sequences (method 2) showed that for each pair there were fewer observed responses than expected given the number of units that occurred in categories 9, 8, and 7. A chi-square test of significance yielded $\chi^2 = 7.33$ ($P \leq .05$); the major deviation from expected values occurred in the 8-5 sequence.

Sequence Analysis

The session was divided into four sequential groups consisting of 106 units each and one final group of 105 units. The total number of units involved in the mutual interactions between C and H, C and W, and C and O (both counselees) are shown in Figure 2.1; these five groups account for 95% of all the units.

The first segment was dominated by W, the second by C, the third and fourth segments by both H and W, and the last, again, by C. Transaction 76 occurred shortly after the beginning of the third segment (i.e., between II and III in Fig. 2.1).

C's direct interactions with H were relatively constant in each part of the session; with W, however, he appeared to be more directively active in the earlier parts of the session than in the later parts of it. Major periods of information provision on C's part occurred in the second and final parts of the session (recall, over 80% of C–O interactions were in the categories 4, 5, and 6).

H showed little involvement in the session except in the third and fourth segments where, compared to the other segments, there was nearly a fivefold increase in verbalizations. W was most active in the initial part of the session, dropping off sharply in the second segment, and then showing an overall increase in the final segments.

Content Analysis

The Bales system involves a scoring method of the process issues in a session, not of its content. To obtain some index of the idiosyncratic content of the session, we proceeded with a quantification of the topical contents within each scored category.

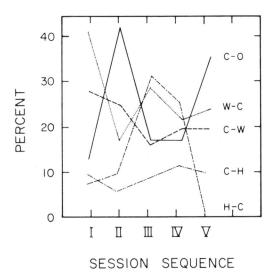

Figure 2.1. *Proportion of units in specified dyadal interactions during the course of a session.*

First, we excluded from the analysis units that consisted of colloquial expressions (e.g., "as far as we know," "you know," "I mean," etc.). This reduced the total number of units from 529 to 433, which were distributed as follows: C, 214 units; W, 142 units; and H, 77 units.

Figure 2.2 shows the distribution of the units of the participants arranged according to their topical content.

In the units originating from the counselees, 42.5% involved expressions of feelings, anxieties, personal opinions, and information about life expectancies and events that preceded the meeting with the counselor. This included statements about their marriage, their experiences as adoptive parents, the meaning of the present pregnancy, and concerns about their personal health status.

In 47.5% of the units originating from the counselees, personal opinions, anxieties, reflections, and feelings were expressed concerning the informational content of the session relative to their immediate future life. This included statements about abortion, amniocentesis, Down syndrome, and mental retardation.

In 10% of the counselees' units, they expressed doubts and opinions, and asked questions about the counselor's role and about the reasons for the counseling; only 19.0% of their total meaningful units were requests for factual information.

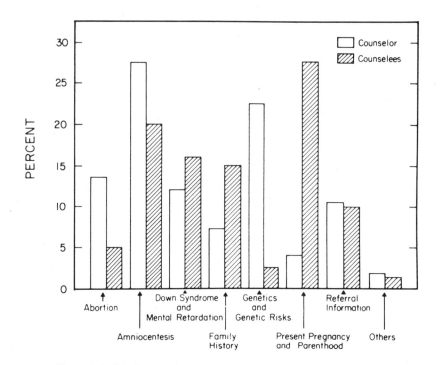

Figure 2.2. Distribution of content issues in a genetic counseling session.

For C, 10.7% of his units concerned the reasons for the counseling session and his personal role. Obtaining medical history comprised 11.7% of his units; 75.7% of the units consisted of providing factual information regarding abortion, amniocentesis, genetic risks, Down syndrome, and mental retardation; 1.9% concerned the couple's decision about having the amniocentesis procedure. Only 14.5% of his meaningful units were questions directed toward the counselees and these consisted largely of requests for factual information.

TEST OF HYPOTHESIS

Hypothesis 1

This hypothesis states that C's counseling style was content-oriented, implying that his interactions with the counselees tended to significantly favor attention to factual information rather than to affective and expressive material and process issues. To test this hypothesis, it was necessary to develop an operational definition of content-orientation. Given the nature of genetic counseling and the role of genetic education in it, it is highly likely that virtually every session would show a major focus on the provision of factual information. This might also be true of sessions in which genetic counseling is psychologically oriented and in which the information might subserve different ends than those in the content-oriented sessions. However, it might be possible to operationalize counseling styles by postulating that genetic counseling sessions would show a balance between instrumental and expressive issues. It then becomes a matter of deciding at which point a balance demonstrates one style as opposed to another. We have postulated that a twofold difference between factual and informational content on the one hand, and affective and expressive content on the other, is to be expected even in genetic counseling that is psychologically oriented. After removal of colloquialisms and other units that might tend to inflate the units in category 6, such as those provided in the course of expansive genetic education (e.g., transactions 55 and 59), if a significant excess beyond a twofold difference is found, this will be taken as evidence of a content-oriented counseling style.

The hypothesis can be tested by comparing the units in categories 7 and 6 (initiated by C), which concern requests for and provision of information, to those in categories 8 and 5, which involve, respectively, requests for and provision of attitudes and feelings. If the sum of the units in categories 7 and 6 significantly exceed the sum of the units in categories 8 and 5 by a factor of 2, this will be taken as evidence of a content-oriented rather than a psychologically oriented style of counseling. In the present case, the excess is more than fourfold and the departure from expected values is highly significant ($\chi^2 = 19.22$; $P < .001$).

Another index of content-orientation can be derived from the kinds of questions C asked. Two types of questions may be distinguished, based on standard interview techniques (Rasche et al., 1974): *direct* questions, which tend to elicit responses of a limited factual nature (e.g., "How old are your children?"), or one-word responses, and *open-ended* questions, which tend to elicit a broader range of information as well as the counselee's thoughts and formulations. In a content-oriented session, one might expect a preponderance of direct questions.

In the transcript analyzed here, C verbalized 32 questions of which only 21.2% were open-ended and the remainder direct.

Hypothesis 2

This hypothesis relates to the possible differential interactions of C with the two counselees. C's verbalizations were more than twice as frequent toward W than toward H; however, the quality of the interactions differed markedly. Of C's negative responses, 80% were directed at W; none of the latter responses were directed exclusively toward H. An estimate of the quality of the interactions directed respectively toward H and W by C can be obtained by taking the ratio of positive units less negative ones for H and W, separately adjusting for differences in their respective numbers of responses. If the ratio, [H] (A − D/A + D)/[W](A − D/A + D) is significantly greater than unity, it would indicate that the quality of interactions toward H was more positive (and less negative) than toward W. If the ratio is less than unity, the reverse would be true. The ratio was calculated to +6.3, suggesting that C was more negative toward W than toward H and that the net result was a relatively greater positive response to H than to W. The number of C–H and C–W units in categories 1 and 12 were compared by means of Fisher's exact test and found to be significantly different ($P \leq 0.05$). The content of the rewards given to the two counselees also differed. When the direct rewards were divided into three groups, personal rewards, formal rewards, and rewards in which reassurance and elevation of status occurred, all five personal rewards went to H, all four rewards with status-raising content went to H, and six out of the seven formal rewards went to W.

Hypothesis 3

This hypothesis states that transaction 76 marked a turning point in the session in which the quality of the interactions between the participants changed significantly. This hypothesis can be evaluated by comparing the interactions prior and subsequent to transaction 76 for the following characteristics:

1. An increase or decrease of overall units originating from one or more participants, or between one or more pairs of participants.
2. An increase or decrease of units in specific categories.

To test the hypothesis, we restricted the analysis to the 100 units immediately preceding transaction 76, and an equal number of units following it, excluding transaction 76 from the analysis. The number, 100, was chosen simply for its convenience in analysis.

Table 2.3 shows the distribution of the 100 unit scores preceding and the 100 scores following transaction 76; this transaction has been excluded. Preceding transaction 76,

Table 2.3. Distribution of Attribution Scores in the 100 Units, Preceding Transaction 76 and the 100 Units Following

		1	2	3	4	5	6	7	8	9	10	11	12	Total
C–H:	Pre	0	0	0	0	0	1	0	0	0	0	0	0	1
	Post	5	0	1	1	1	2	0	1	0	0	0	0	11
C–W:	Pre	5	0	0	6	3	23	0	0	0	0	0	3	40
	Post	0	0	0	0	2	2	0	0	0	0	0	0	4
C–O:	Pre	1	0	0	5	0	31	1	0	0	0	0	0	38
	Post	0	0	0	0	2	12	2	3	0	0	0	0	19
H–C:	Pre	0	0	0	0	0	0	0	0	0	0	0	0	0
	Post	0	1	0	0	7	24	1	1	0	0	2	0	36
H–W:	Pre	0	0	0	0	0	0	0	0	0	0	0	0	0
	Post	0	0	0	0	0	1	0	0	0	0	0	0	1
H–O:	Pre	0	0	0	0	0	0	0	0	0	0	0	0	0
	Post	0	0	0	0	0	0	0	0	0	0	0	0	0
W–C:	Pre	0	0	1	0	2	5	10	0	0	0	1	2	21
	Post	0	0	0	0	7	16	2	0	0	0	0	1	26
W–H:	Pre	0	0	0	0	0	0	0	0	0	0	0	0	0
	Post	0	0	0	0	0	0	0	0	0	2	0	0	2
W–O:	Pre	0	0	0	0	0	0	0	0	0	0	0	0	0
	Post	0	0	0	0	0	0	0	0	0	0	0	0	1
Total	pre	6	0	1	11	5	60	11	0	0	0	1	5	
Total	post	5	1	1	1	20	57	5	5	0	2	2	1	
Total		11	1	2	12	25	117	16	5	0	2	3	6	200

C = counselor, H = husband, W = wife, O = both.

C clearly dominated the interactions; he originated 79% of the units; H contributed none. Following transaction 76, C's contributions declined 58.3% and the number of units originating from the counselees increased over 260%; in particular, H became noticeably more verbal.

Most conspicuous is a significant increase of verbal interactions across categories between C and H ($\chi^2 = 8.40$; $P < .01$) and vice versa, and a significant decrease ($\chi^2 = 15.10$; $P < .001$) of verbal interactions with W.

Since transaction 76 emphasized attitudes and feelings preferentially to information and orientation, it might be expected that to the extent the intervention affected the participants, an increase of units in categories 5 and 8 relative to units in categories 6 and 7 might follow the transaction. The pre- and post-scores of units in categories 5 and 8 were compared to those in categories 6 and 7 and found to be significantly increased ($\chi^2 = 11.8$; $P < .001$).

Hypothesis 4

According to the Bales system, categories 9 and 4 might provide information on the directiveness and control exerted by the participants. We are particularly interested in the number of instances of control and directiveness shown by C; all 18 units scored in category 4 were attributed to C in the present transcript. These units can be divided into four groups:

1. routinely accepts control within the session itself (7 units);
2. orients the other's attention (5 units);
3. influences the other's evaluations of genetic risk rates (5 units);
4. advises the counselees regarding the use of excess amniotic fluid (1 unit).

There are only three units scored in category 9; all initiated by W. These are as follows:

Transaction 122: "Do most women have them aborted when they know they're like this?" This question, directed to C, follows not long after he has shown the counselees a picture of a Down syndrome child (transaction 60). In reply to the question, C said: "A lot of people have. Some people decided, they have strong feelings about abortion, and have decided not to go ahead with the abortion. . . ."

Transaction 171: "Do you?" (W to H): This question, posed to C, regarded the giving of permission for the use of excess amniotic fluid for research purposes.

Transaction 173: "What do most people put?" This question, posed to C, regarded the giving of permission for the use of excess amniotic fluid. C replied, "They usually say, yeah."

In only one of these instances, the last, did C *directly* provide advice regarding the counselees' actions. The reply dealing with abortion does not contain explicit directive or specific action. It did, however, contain normative information and, hence, an implied message of appropriate action. However, the reply is so complex that it merits further attention—more than can be given at this juncture.

DISCUSSION

Several methods have been used to study the interactions that occur in the professional–client or "more-knowing–less-knowing" relationship. Bales (1950) developed a 12-point scoring system to study small group interactions along two dimensions, a cognitive-affective dimension with positive and negative aspects and a task-oriented one with instrumental and expressive aspects. Flanders (1966) developed a 10-point scale consisting of an analysis of initiation and response characteristics in pupil–teacher interactions. Byrne and Long (1976) studied doctor–patient interactions by scoring behaviors in three domains: doctor-centered, patient-centered, and negative behaviors.

The Bales system has been used to study physician–patient interactions with a focus on compliance (Davis, 1968) as well as on the overall quality of doctor–patient communication (Korsch and Negrete, 1972). Because it appears to focus on problem-solving strategies, the Bales system was attractive for use in scoring transcripts of genetic counseling sessions, where task-oriented and problem-solving issues are major components.

From the previous qualitative analysis of the transcript (Kessler, 1981 and this volume), four hypotheses emerged. These were tested by means of the data derived from the quantitative analysis. It was possible to confirm three of the hypotheses. The fourth one, dealing with counselor directiveness, was difficult to either confirm or disconfirm using this system of analysis. A more detailed analysis of this problem will be reported elsewhere.

Hypothesis 1 dealt with the issue of C's content-oriented style of counseling. An attempt was made to make content-oriented counseling operational by assuming that factual information will virtually always be the predominant focus of genetic counseling, even when the psychosocial issues are attended to, but that content-orientation would occur when the number of units of factual information significantly exceeded more than twice the number of units of attitudinal and affective content. It is recognized that this definition and the cutoff point involved have been arbitrarily chosen. However, in the absence of precedents, or models, it was felt that despite possible deficiencies our definition is heuristic and open to further tests in future research.

In the present analysis, the hypothesis was confirmed. Factual information was attended to four times more frequently than attitudinal and affective material. The analysis of the topical content of this session confirmed our process analysis; more than three-quarters of the unit content originating from C dealt with factual information.

Hypothesis 2 stated that C behaved differently toward the two counselees, mostly positive toward H and negatively toward W. This was studied by comparing the relative number of "reward" (category 1) and "punishments" or acts of aggression (category 12) meted out to each by C. The difference was found to be significant and the hypothesis confirmed. These findings might have been idiosyncratic to this C and/or this session. However, the possibility that this may represent a more general aspect of couples work in genetic counseling needs to be explored, since it may affect the overall effectiveness of the counseling, the satisfaction derived from it by the participants, and the later interpersonal processes of the counselees.

Hypothesis 3 related to the effects of a specific intervention (transaction 76) on the subsequent course of the session. This intervention occurred following the taking of a health and family history and the presentation of an age-appropriate risk figure for Down syndrome by C. He stated that "a woman your age has about a 2% chance of having a child with any chromosomal disorder." To which W replied, "Especially when it's the first one after 22 years of marriage." C had a choice at this point. On one hand, he might have corrected W's mistaken belief that her risk for a child with a chromosomal abnormality was a function of the fact that she was primigravida; this would have been consistent with the counseling approach he had used up to that point, namely, a focus on content and factual material. On the other hand, he could choose to reply to the underlying meaning or metamessage (Kessler, 1979b) of W's statement, which emphasized how important the pregnancy was for her. In choosing the latter course, it is suggested that the choice the had important consequences in the session. H became more involved in the session and the proportion of expressions of feelings and attitudes increased significantly.

It could be argued that the changes detected here might have been the consequence of some other of C's interventions or of a statement emanating from the counselees prior to or immediately following the index transaction. Quantitative analysis cannot rule out these possibilities; qualitative analysis of the transcript is a more powerful guide in this regard. The quality of C's statements at transaction 76 differed so markedly from whatever was said prior to this point, that it seems unlikely that other statements and events in the session can account for the changes that occurred. One might speculate that by focusing attention on the issue raised by W in the previous transaction (75), C might have signaled his readiness to hear and discuss an issue raised earlier in the session by the counselees, and about which they appeared to be eager to talk.

The Bales analysis did not shed much light on the problem of counselor directiveness. In all, there were three instances of requests for advice or direction from the counselees and in only one did C give direct advice. This involved a situation in which abortion or reproduction were not issues. In regard to abortion, C was asked what most couples do after a fetus with a chromosomal abnormality is detected. C's reply included normative information that may have conveyed an implied directive as to what course the counselees ought to follow. We have concluded at this point that there is insufficient information derived from the quantitative analysis to either confirm or disconfirm that C was directive.

The data of this study suggest that the Bales system is a promising one for further analyses and/or comparisons of other genetic counseling transcripts. It might be useful to point out some of the strengths and limitations of this scoring system. The power of the Bales system is that it restricts the assignment of category scores of units in relation to the units either immediately proximal or distal to them. This leads to a maximizing of inter-rater reliability in the independent scoring of the transcript material. However, this also leads to the loss of important information regarding the context in which the unit occurs. Since it is the context that ultimately gives the unit its particular meaning (Mishler, 1979), a loss of contextual information may reduce the generalities one might draw from the data. The application of both qualitative and quantitative analyses of transcripts may be the only way to resolve this dilemma.

The present study demonstrates the feasibility of applying quantitative methods to elucidate the process of genetic counseling. This opens the way for further study of different styles of counseling for the same (or similar) genetic disorders and comparative studies of counseling for differing genetic disorders. Such investigations may identify within-session process variables contributing in major ways to later outcome measures of effectiveness and satisfaction. Also, it may be possible to study the effects of specific interventions related to the process of genetic education (e.g., how a recurrence risk is stated) or the psychological issues (e.g., alleviation of guilt) on short-term (within session) and long-term (postcounseling) consequences. In addition, how psychosocial issues in general and such specific issues as directiveness are dealt with in the genetic counseling session can be investigated to identify effective and ineffective approaches. In sum, further study of process variables may provide information that could promote more effective genetic counseling and facilitate the training of genetic counselors.

ACKNOWLEDGMENTS

We are grateful to Dr. Everett Dempster for his statistical advice and to Ms. Martha Raftery for typing the final draft of the manuscript.

REFERENCES

Antley MA, Antley RM, Hartlage LC (1973) Effects of genetic counseling on parental self-concepts. J Psychol 83:335–338.

Antley RM, Hartlage LC (1976) Psychological responses to genetic counseling for Down's syndrome. Clin Genet 9:257–265.

Bales RF (1950) Interaction Process Analysis. Cambridge, MA: Addison-Wesley Press.

Black RB (1979) The effect of diagnostic uncertainty and available options on perceptions of risk. Birth Defects: Original Article Series (5C):341–354.

Byrne PS, Long BEL (1976) Doctors Talking to Patients. London: Her Majesty's Stationery Office.

Carter CO, Roberts JAF, Evans KA, Buck AR (1971) Genetic clinic: a follow-up. Lancet 1:281–285.

Childs B (1978) Genetic counseling: a critical review of the published literature. In: Cohen BH, Lilienfeld AM, Huang PC (eds). Genetic Issues in Public Health and Medicine. Springfield, IL: CC Thomas, pp 329–357.

Corgan RL (1979) Genetic counseling and parental self-concept. Birth Defects: Original Article Series 15(5C):281–285.

Davis MS (1968) Variations in patients' compliance with doctors' advice: an empirical analysis of patterns of communications. Am J Public Health 58:274–288.

Emery AEH, Watt MS, Clark ER (1972) The effects of genetic counseling in Duchenne muscular dystrophy. Clin Genet 3:147–150.

Flanders NA (1966) Interaction Analysis in the Classroom: A Manual for Observers. Ann Arbor: University of Michigan Press.

Hsia YE (1977) Approaches to the appraisal of genetic counseling. In: Lubs H, de la Cruz F (eds). Genetic Counseling. New York: Academic Press, pp 17–33.

Kessler S (1979a) The psychological foundations of genetic counseling. In: Kessler S (ed). Genetic Counseling: Psychological Dimensions. New York: Academic Press, pp 35–51.

Kessler S (1979b) The processes of communication, decision making and coping in genetic counseling. In: Kessler S (ed). Genetic Counseling: Psychological Dimensions. New York: Academic Press, pp 137–153.

Kessler S (1981) Psychological aspects of genetic counseling: analysis of a transcript. Am J Med Genet 8:137–153.

Korchin SJ (1976) Modern Clinical Psychology. New York: Basic Books.

Korsch BM, Negrete VF (1972) Doctor–patient communication. Sci Am 277:66–74.

Leonard CO, Chase GA, Childs B (1972) Genetic counseling: a consumer's view. N Engl J Med 287:433–439.

Lubs ML (1979) Does genetic counseling influence risk attitudes and decision making? Birth Defects: Original Article Series 15(5C):355–367.

Mishler EG (1979) Meaning in context: is there any other kind? Harvard Educ Rev 49:1–19.

Rasche LM, Berstein L, Veenhuis PE (1974) Evaluation of a systematic approach to teaching interviewing. J Med Educ 49:589–595.

Reynolds BD, Puck MH, Robinson A (1974) Genetic counseling: an appraisal. Clin Genet 5:177–187.

Rowley PT, Fisher L, Lipkin M (1979) Screening and genetic counseling for β-thalassemia trait in a population unselected for interest: effects on knowledge and mood. Am J Hum Genet 31:718–730.

Shaw M (1977) Review of published studies of genetic counseling: a critique of methodology. In: Lubs H, de la Cruz F (eds). Genetic Counseling. New York: Raven Press, pp 35–49.

Sibinga MS, Friedman CJ (1971) Complexities of parental understanding of phenylketonuria. Pediatrics 48:216–224.

Siegel S (1956) Nonparametric Statistics for the Behavioral Sciences. New York: McGraw-Hill Book Co.

Sorenson JR, Swazey JP, Scotch NS (1980) Impact of genetic counseling: results of the collaborative study. Paper presented at Birth Defects Conference, New York City, June 11, 1980.

3

Management of Guilt and Shame[1]

INTRODUCTION

The birth of a child with a genetic or congenital defect is frequently associated with thoughts and feelings of guilt and shame in the parents. These psychological responses are observed frequently in genetic counseling as parents review historical details and struggle to find reasons, causes, and meaning in the occurrence of the defect. The ascription of personal responsibility in such circumstances is a normal response to events over which the person generally has little or no control and with it the concomitant sense that the future occurrence of personal pain and hurt will be averted. Shame, too, is a common response to situations in which one feels that personal deficiencies or failures are exposed, as they are when one perceives one's imperfect reproductive products.

Guilt and shame reactions consist of interrelated cognitive, affective, behavioral, and, sometimes, obvious physiological components. The reactions may be of relatively short duration, as, for example, the blush of embarrassment. On the other hand, they may persist for relatively long periods of time, penetrating and influencing areas of the person's functioning, apparently unrelated to the stimuli that evoked these states originally.

Genetic counselors frequently need to deal with guilt and/or shame states during the course of genetic counseling (Hecht and Holmes, 1972), and in many ways, they are in a unique position to do so. Parents of children born with congenital malformations and/or genetic disorders frequently seek for causal connections between the

---

[1]This essay first appeared as Kessler S, Kessler H, Ward P (1984) Psychological aspects of genetic counseling. III. Management of guilt and shame. *American Journal of Medical Genetics* 17:673–697. Reprinted with kind permission of the publisher, John Wiley and Sons.

defect and prior thoughts, fantasies, wishes, and/or actions. When their attributions are unrealistic, new information obtained in the course of genetic counseling may diminish feelings of guilt and shame. Furthermore, genetic counselors may be among the first or only professional to whom guilt and/or shame responses are revealed by many persons. Thus, the genetic counseling interaction may be the one and only opportunity for a professional to intervene and modify the beliefs and feelings connected with these reactions. Also, genetic counselors often see counselees at times and in situations when the latter may be relatively open to suggestions that may have a long-lasting impact on their cognitive and affective functioning. Appropriate comments and suggestions may facilitate the process of genetic education, and, presumably, increase the chances of later adaptive behavior and rational decision making. Such counseling interventions[2] would also prime counselees for effective counseling or therapy later on and/or promote subsequent productive psychological work. On the other hand, inappropriate or ineffective interventions may have the opposite effect and make it more difficult for the counselees to utilize other counseling professionals to best advantage. In this regard, the lack of appropriate comments on the counselee's guilt or shame, when called for, may, in itself, be an inappropriate intervention.

Although the reduction of guilt or shame is a worthy goal, virtually no guidelines exist in the genetic counseling literature by means of which this goal might be accomplished. The apparently common practice of simply telling people that they did nothing about which they should feel guilty has struck us as being an immensely oversimplified and, in some cases, a counterproductive strategy for dealing with the complexities and myriad forms of the guilt and shame reactions encountered in genetic counseling. If the person's dominant state is one of shame rather than of guilt, this particular approach may be ineffective or inappropriate. Also, there are instances and actions for which the maintenance rather than the alleviation of guilt feelings would be a more appropriate counseling aim.

As a prophylactic measure some genetic counselors tell many of their counselees almost routinely that persons like themselves frequently feel guilty about having a child with a genetic problem, but that it was something over which they had no control, that is, it was a chance event. In our experience, such statements are not effective, as little or no prior exploration is made of the counselees' inner experience and beliefs and the statement may not directly address the content of the counselees' feelings. In our view, effective counseling interventions need to be based on an accurate assessment of the kind and quality of guilt or shame the counselee displays. The predominant state, guilt or shame, needs to be identified and an assessment made of its content and developmental level of elaboration; cultural and existential issues may need to be taken into account. Also, in planning and making appropriate interventions, the psychological defenses of the counselees need to be assessed as well as the counselee's readiness for specific suggestions.

In this paper we will consider guilt and shame reactions. First, we will differentiate these reactions and point out some of the psychological defenses and develop-

---

[2]Counseling interventions refer to the counselor's attempts to focus the counselees' attention and, explicitly or implicity, suggest new or different ways of thinking and assessing one's experience

mental issues associated with each. Then, we will consider how each might be manifested in genetic counseling. Finally, we will suggest the kinds of interventions that might be made to alleviate their distressing aspects.

GUILT AND SHAME DIFFERENTIATED

The concepts of guilt and shame are frequently confused and the two states are sometimes collapsed into a single concept, guilt (Lewis, 1971). In the psychoanalytic literature, guilt is generally associated with responses of self-reproach to violations of *internalized* standards, whereas shame is frequently associated with responses to anticipated or actual *external* disapproval, ridicule, and scorn. Piers and Singer (1953) suggest that guilt arises out of a tension between the so-called ego and superego functions whereas shame arises out of a tension between ego and ego ideal. According to this view, the concept of *superego* might be thought of as encompassing two distinct functions: (1) that of an internalized monitoring agency by which personal behavior is evaluated and judged and (2) that of an ego ideal, the totality of positive identifications with parental images and ideals. Guilt arises when the internal monitoring agency "informs" the ego that one of its rules has been violated, whereas feelings of shame arise when one's behavior falls short of an internalized ideal of what one's behavior should be and the discrepancy is thought to be visible to all. These superego functions are believed to develop through processes of identification involving, in the case of guilt, the incorporation of strictures and implied threats associated with oedipal issues (e.g., castration) and, in the case of shame, identification follows the first route of imitation and them the emulation of admired others.

To put the matter more simply, guilt might be thought of as arising from transgressions of prohibitions, whereas shame arises from failures to reach goals and ideals (Piers and Singer, 1953; Lynd, 1958). In guilt reactions, individuals hold themselves responsible for some negatively perceived outcome or consequence, the transgression constituting an act of commission or of omission, thoughts, wishes, and so on. Since one is responsible for the outcome, negative self-evaluations follow, including the belief that one is punishable.

Guilt may either be realistic or unrealistic. In the former, the person had the capacity to influence the outcome as, for example, in the case of a man who had a Down syndrome child after asking his wife not to have an amniocentesis even though it was offered to and preferred by her. In unrealistic guilt, the person assumes responsibility for the negative outcomes regardless of their ability to control the factors influencing the outcome. This often happens around reproductive issues where one almost invariably has little control over the final product. However, people generally act as if chance processes were not operating and as if they had—or should have had—control over the outcome. Since the ability to exercise control over one's primary functions (including reproductive ones) is an important element in one's ego ideal, the feeling of loss of control that occurs in assuming unrealistic responsibility may evoke not only feelings of guilt, but also those of shame.

Feelings of shame are related to the self-system (see below). In contrast to guilt, shame is a relatively more psychologically passive state, often associated with feelings of inadequacy and helplessness in which the failure to live up to the ego ideal triggers a loss of self-esteem and feelings of unworthiness. The diminution of one's self-worth is experienced as a "narcissistic injury."

There are differing degrees of shame, ranging from chagrin and embarrassment, on one hand, to humiliation and mortification, on the other. But in all shame reactions, the mechanism is the same, that is, the internalized ego ideal is *projected* outward and on to external objects, the ubiquitous "they." This process of projection or externalization is what renders one helpless and passive because it is not felt that one has control over the evaluations of the "other." Therefore, shame is experienced in relationship with the "world," that is, how others will think about, feel about, and judge you. In other words, in how they will "see" you. Therefore, shame tends to be experienced in terms of visual imagery and in autonomic reactions and, relative to guilt, has little or poorly elaborated cognitive content. The visual aspects are expressed or experienced in terms of feeling exposed, wanting to avert one's eyes, wanting to hide out of sight, etc., and are generally associated with relatively prominent affective reactions. Guilt, on the other hand, may or may not be involved with overt affective reactions (Lewis, 1971) and cognitive aspects tend to be relatively elaborated. For example, guilt is often associated with well-developed systems of belief, with or without rational foundation, regarding cause–effect relationships and one's personal role in an attributory chain.

DEFENSES ASSOCIATED WITH GUILT AND SHAME

Guilt and shame tend to be associated with different psychological defense mechanisms. As we pointed out, shame tends to be experienced in wanting to hide or hide away from the eyes of a judging world the issues or problems that are believed to be the source of the shame. In order to protect oneself from the judgment of others or bolster one's self-esteem one might:

1. deny that anything is wrong (denial), that is, alter external reality by disregarding the presence of the cause of one's loss of self-esteem;
2. invert reality by relabeling a loss as a gain (reaction formation), for example, feeling that one is blessed by having been given the responsibility or opportunity of raising a defective child;
3. find something else to boast or brag about (compensation);
4. find fault with others, thus shifting the spotlight to someone else's deficiencies rather than one's own (displacement).

In guilt reactions, some of the defenses commonly encountered are:

1. personal behaviors for which one might be held accountable may be forgotten (repression);

2. blame for causing the problem may be externalized and personal responsibility diminished by finding "good" reasons and excuses (intellectualization and rationalization);

3. attempts may be made to separate feelings, particularly guilt affect, from thoughts about events (isolation) so that personal "badness" is kept within bounds.

In addition, guilt feelings may themselves be used as a defense against a more intense, albeit covert, sense of shame. For example, the mother of a defective child who takes on a martyr role, irrationally absorbing and accepting full responsibility for the child's problems and care, may be repressing her feelings of disappointment, rejection, and shame while simultaneously purging her guilt feelings through her behavior.

The defensive maneuvers employed to deal with guilt or shame are means by which individuals protect themselves from being overwhelmed by the emotions associated with these states and attempt to maintain their self-esteem. When the defenses leave the person in an emotionally more vulnerable position than previously or less equipped to deal with the reality of their situation, then it might be desirable for the counselor to assist the individual to find more adaptive protective postures.

DEVELOPMENTAL ISSUES

The degree to which guilt is differentiated appears to be related to the person's level of moral development. Piaget (1948), Kohlberg (1963), and others have suggested that in the course of individual development, moral thinking progresses from one stage to the next depending on corresponding progress in cognitive development. Moral thought is believed to move from *preconventional* to *conventional* to *postconventional* stages. In the first, there is a concern with the avoidance of punishment rather than with following internalized values; acts are evaluated on the basis of consequences rather than intentions and on their instrumental value in meeting egocentric needs, that is, rules are followed only on the basis of personal gain or loss. In *conventional* stages, conformity to fixed rules, authority, and the social order are prominent in the person's thinking; the right thing is what gains approval from others or maintains, rigidly, the existing moral or social order. In *postconventional* stages moral judgments take into account the rights of others and are based solely on transcendent values, and the process of making moral judgments achieves flexibility.

Ruma and Mosher (1967) showed that the stage of moral judgment was significantly correlated to measures of guilt; the more advanced the stage the greater the degree of internalized guilt emotion. The findings suggest that the person's level of thinking about moral issues influences the sophistication and degree of elaboration of guilt cognition. More advanced levels of guilt tend to have an internal cognitive focus in which self-blame, negative self-judgments, and remorse are prominent, whereas less advanced guilt is marked by an external focus in which a fear or thoughts of punishment and retribution may be present. In less advanced levels of guilt, the cognitive focus on the guilt-associated events tends to be nonspecific and global with little or no indication that mitigating circumstances may have played a role. Self-judgment tends to be severe and the concept of self-compassion appears to be alien or ego-dystonic. In more advanced levels of guilt, the cognitive focus is on a specific guilt-associated event, mitigating circumstances have been considered, and the ideas of penance and forgiveness are in the realm of possibility.

In contrast to guilt, the ontogeny of shame reactions is less well understood. In his discussion of ego development, Erikson (1963) suggests that shame derives from a maturational conflict in early life, whose resolution leads to a sense of autonomy, whereas a resolutional block or failure promotes a sense of shame and doubt in the child. Erikson believes that a central element in this conflict is, on one hand, the *development* of self-control with its attending feelings of high self-esteem and pride and, on the other, a *loss* of self-control or the assignment of control to external agents (such as one's parents) or other authority figures leading to doubt in one's own abilities to exert control and one's self-worth. This leaves the person with a propensity to be shamed.

Current psychodynamic thinking emphasizes that one's ability to evaluate and assess one's worth realistically is subject to developmental and learning processes. These learning processes normally include interactions with parents and other important adults in which it is learned that one is valuable (narcissism) and that others are to be valued in turn. For some persons, the learning about the self is faulty, leading to pervasive tendencies to misregulate the self-evaluative processes. These individuals tend to either overevaluate (leading to states of grandiosity) or to underestimate (leading to depressive states) one's self worth. Misregulation may occur after an ego loss or the threat of a loss has occurred; the threat may be the result of a personal insult, a perceived lack of empathy on the part of "powerful" others, etc.

When one's capacity to regulate one's self-esteem is faulty or poorly developed, the tendency is to look to others, particularly to perceived powerful others, and to externals (e.g., sports cars, diamonds, possessions, etc.) as a source of maintaining or bolstering one's self-esteem. Thus, persons with self-esteem regulatory difficulties tend to idealize physicians, counselors, and other perceived authority figures and to show a strongly marked need to be seen in a good light by others (Kohut, 1971). Such persons are particularly affected by the occurrence of birth and genetic defects.

Like guilt reactions, those of shame might also be divided developmentally into relatively less advanced and more advanced forms on the basis of the degree of affective intensity and the kind of focus displayed by the person. In the more advanced forms of shame, the affective intensity tends to be contained and the focus is more internal or self-oriented, whereas in less advanced forms of shame, affective intensity tends to be high and the focus is less well articulated and global.

Less advanced shame tends to be marked by rage and other intense reactions or relatively extreme hiding behavior. In more advanced shame, the affective response and associated behaviors are more moderated and the compensating behaviors are more realistic. Whereas in more advanced shame a child's defects might be hidden as, for example, in letting the hair grow long to cover a malformed ear; in less advanced shame, the child may be hidden away. One might also see the compensatory opposite of hiding, which in an extreme form might be marked by boastful or exhibitionist behavior, in which the defect is elevated to a status or sign of superiority over normal individuals.

GUILT AND SHAME REACTIONS IN THE CONTEXT OF GENETIC COUNSELING

From the onset, we would like to suggest that much of what comes to be labeled as guilt, in the genetic counseling situation, may actually be shame reactions. The birth of a child with a genetic or congenital defect is generally experienced as a narcissistic wound (Kessler, 1979a; Targum, 1981) with concomitant feelings of diminished self-esteem and a loss of control. Parents normally invest of themselves (narcissistic investment) in a pregnancy. If the pregnancy leads to joy and fulfillment, the parents feel pride in themselves and are proud of their child. However, if the pregnancy leads to disappointment or despair, the parents are likely to feel a sense of failure and experience shame.

If a couple is singled out and advised that they require special attention and counseling around future reproductive decisions and behavior over which most others normally exert autonomous control, then this might be experienced as a sign of deficiency, triggering feelings of shame. The threat of discovering a defect inherent in such prenatal diagnostic procedures as amniocentesis is sometimes experienced with shame or anticipated shame (see Example 7, below). The need to consider, in advance, a decision to abort a genetically defective fetus may underscore the possibility that one might not or cannot produce a normal child, and hence one is inherently deficient. In short, the potential for a defect in one's products reflects negatively on one's own inherent worth leading to shame reactions. Such reactions may be displayed in a tendency toward "no shows" or repeated cancellations of appointments, affective shutdown, or expression of anger, the latter sometimes being above and beyond what one might reasonably expect from the situation. Counselees who are unusually belligerent, difficult to counsel, threatening (litigation, among other things), and who otherwise make the counselor defensive or angry, may, we believe, experience or perceive the (actual or potential) genetic defect as a narcissistic wound, that is, as an attack on the self-esteem, and hence display shame reactions.

Persons with narcissistic deficiencies, whose self-esteem is labile and fragile, are particularly vulnerable when a genetic diagnosis occurs. This may trigger unusual rage reactions or hyperactivity generally in the service of undoing the narcissistic wound by proving the diagnosis or diagnostician wrong, or depressive reactions.

Because reproductive decisions involve sexual thoughts, actions, and feelings, the area of reproduction is frequently associated with feelings of guilt and shame. Decisions to delay further reproduction or to have a "replacement" child quickly following a stillborn or early death of a child with a defect might be interpreted as strategies to deal with feelings of guilt or shame. The production of a healthy child following narcissistic injury or devalued self-worth that attends the birth of one with a defect is an attempt to repair one's lowered self-esteem.

A frequent situation that emerges in preamniocentesis counseling is one in which the counselees have not informed their family, relatives, or friends that "they" are pregnant. Without implying that all such cases can be accounted for by invoking shame dynamics, such dynamics may nevertheless be operating in many instances. These might be understood as a means of dealing with the anticipated shame or humiliation that might occur if the fetus proved to be defective. Thus, the possibility of shame in the near future may be shaping the current behavior of "hiding."

Guilt reactions frequently emerge in the course of genetic counseling around several contexts. When counselees show an unusually intense interest in the genesis of their child's defects, it generally serves more than a search for causes. Often involved is a desire to absolve oneself of responsibility or identity and affix blame elsewhere. When a disorder is transmitted via a dominant or X-linked mode of inheritance, it tends to facilitate the ascription of blame and reinforces the sense of guilt in the "blamed" parent.

In discussing the origin of a child's defects or in the course of obtaining a pregnancy history, the counselees might display confessional needs, sometimes providing the counselor with a long litany of supposed wrongs done in the past, which are now associated with the defects. These indications of guilt may be associated with such other indicators of guilt as statements of disappointment, disapproval, or regret concerning one's commitments, decisions, and behavior. For example, the counselee might say something along the lines of, "I know I shouldn't have had sexual relations the day before my wife was to give birth."

Another major context around which guilt emerges is in the discussion of reproduction and reproductive decisions. Statements such as, "How can I bring another monster into the world?" are indicators of an underlying sense of guilt that generally requires further exploration. A common way of expiating guilt feelings generated by the birth of a child with a genetic defect is to disallow oneself further reproduction.

Some of the guilt reactions seen in the context of genetic counseling are iatrogenic. In their zeal for thoroughness or because of the need to complete family history forms, genetic counselors sometimes ask for and obtain historical data that may have little or no relevance to the particular case under discussion. For example, asking questions of parents with newborn infants with trisomies about their history of drug use or alcohol consumption might suggest to the parents that there is a connection between their past drug-related behavior and the current problem, and that they are responsible, through commission or omission, for their child's problems. If, later on in the session, the counselor says to them that they did nothing to feel guilty about, the parents might be somewhat confused and disbelieving.

A frequent occurrence of iatrogenically induced guilt in genetic counseling follows the undermining of unrealistic attributory beliefs (see Example 1, below). Humans have the need to make causal attributions between their experiences and antecedent factors (Harvey and Smith, 1977). Where the array of informational possibilities is restricted or where defensive motivation may be present, attributional errors are likely to be made. Thus, a common situation in genetic counseling is for counselees to ask such questions as, "Do you think those aspirins I took had something to do with the birth defect in the child?" In most cases there is little or no known relationship between the antecedent events or reactions and the fact of the defect(s); fetal alcohol syndrome is the notable exception. Frequently, the counselor discounts the counselee's attributions in an attempt to correct misinformation. But this does not always lead to productive outcomes. For example, after a series of such discounting statements, the counselee may say, "Well, I guess if it's not those things, it must be me." In such situations, the counselee may have been hoping that the counselor would confirm that some external cause was operative. By undermining this hope or wish, the counselor may be communicating the message that, "You are to blame."

Feelings of guilt tend to increase when the circumstances surrounding the cause and nature of the defect are ambiguous. Thus, when the diagnosis or recurrence risks are uncertain, or when a newly arisen mutation cannot be differentiated from a nongenetic cause, or when incomplete penetrance and variable expressivity are issues, as they frequently are in dominantly inherited disorders, thoughts of self-blame and guilt tend to be promoted. Such thoughts may be reinforced by the general tendency to assign blame and responsibility to the person in ambiguous situations (Jones et al., 1961).

In real life, guilt and shame reactions are often intermixed; Lewis (1971) and Piers and Singer (1953) discuss cycles of guilt and shame. When, out of shame, anger is expressed at another or blame is assigned to another, guilt reactions may follow. Conversely, guilt feelings may be experienced with shame reactions.

The factors that evoke guilt and shame reactions may differ from those that maintain such states over time. The birth of a child with a genetic disease may trigger guilt feelings, but, after several years of unresolved feelings, one needs to wonder about the factors that prevent resolution. Personality factors may be involved. However, frequently the counselor needs to evaluate the role of marital dysfunctions and communication and other interpersonal difficulties in sustaining guilt feelings.

INTERVENTIONS AND CASE ILLUSTRATIONS

In planning and making appropriate counseling interventions, the genetic counselor needs to make an accurate assessment as to which state, guilt or shame, predominates, the quality of the particular state, the level of its elaboration, and the client's response-readiness and overall needs. Following some general remarks regarding counseling tactics directed at guilt and shame, we will present a series of case illustrations in which these psychological reactions occur. Each case will be discussed in terms of its emotional and dynamic meaning and of the specific comments or suggestions made or attempted. Where possible, suggestions will be made regarding alternative interventions that would be appropriate under circumstances similar to those illustrated.

There are several well-known and traditionally effective methods to relieve the distressing aspects of guilt and shame. These are:

1. confession, generally a public acknowledgment of wrongdoing;
2. contrition, more or less a motivation to make amends and redress wrongs; and

3. penance, acts of righting wrongs, and redress with or without accompanying punishment of previous wrongs.

The key step in helping a person deal with feelings of guilt or shame is that of confession in which the person expresses the belief that the undesired outcome is due to a personal act of commission or omission. The belief may have little or no rational justification, yet its verbalization by the counselee is an essential starting point. Thus, the initial counseling strategy leading to a reduction of guilt or shame needs to be the provision of help so that the counselees freely express their beliefs and perceptions about their role in causing the problem that brings them to genetic counseling. When the counselor interferes with or omits the step of confession, it generally reduces the effectiveness of later guilt- or shame-reducing interventions. Frequently, the interference occurs when the counselor prematurely employs *normalizing* tactics (see below) or preempts the counselee's confession by saying, "Many people in your position feel guilt over having a child with a genetic problem. You need to know that there was nothing you did that caused it." When such well-documented statements precede or prevent confessional work on the part of the counselees, they are generally not helpful.

Guilt involves major cognitive elements, whereas shame is more prominently an affective state. Thus, cognitively oriented interventions may be more effective in relieving guilt than strategies designed to promote affective expression or relief, an approach that may be better suited for long-term therapeutic work rather than genetic counseling. Comments with a high degree of empathy, directed at affective levels of communication, would be suitable for dealing with shame reactions.

Some persons may be more stylistically prone toward guilt rather than toward shame states and vice versa. However, at any given time, one state tends to be the dominant or more obviously manifest one. It is important for the counselor to recognize which state is dominant at any given time, because the different states involve different cognitive processes, which, in turn, lead to different mental sets vis-à-vis the preparation and positioning for later problem solving. This implies that differing counseling approaches may be needed depending on the particular cognitive-affective processes used by the counselee. These processes are both situation specific and a product of life experiences and developmental processes.

GUILT-ALLEVIATING TACTICS

After confession has occurred, several tactics may be employed to relieve guilt feelings:

Use of authority. The counselor uses the full force of their professional role to tell the counselees that they are guiltless. In our experience, such interventions appear more effective when used at or around the time the genetic diagnosis is made rather than later on. When worded appropriately, the counselor's statement serves as a cognitive reference point that can be retrieved or used as a self-reminder when later ideas and thoughts of guilt emerge. This assists the person to mitigate the sting of these later self-recriminations.

Normalization. The counselor points out that others in the counselee's position would feel exactly as they do. The counselor's aim is to reduce the sense of social and psychological isolation, stigmatization, and "specialness" associated with the guilt cognition and to affirm the appropriateness of the counselee's beliefs (see Example 4, below).

Reframing. The counselor helps the counselee acquire a new cognitive frame of reference in which perceptions and actions take on different (and less distressful) meaning. For example, an approach we have used with some success with persons expressing responsibility for a child's birth defects was to confirm that, indeed, the person was responsible. "Indeed, you are responsible, a responsible human being. If you weren't that kind of person you wouldn't be feeling what you are feeling. But, because you are a responsible person doesn't mean you are responsible for the genes you transmitted to your child or for his problems."

Limiting liability. The illustration above also attempts to help the person set limits as to their personal responsibility: "You are responsible for *a* but not for *b*."

In less advanced forms of guilt, defensive operations will probably be operating at a maximum. This keeps the individual from experiencing the full impact of their feelings, and from exploring and examining the experience. Since these processes need to occur before absolution and penance become effective, strategies at relieving or absolving guilt will probably be ineffective. Counseling strategies ought to accentuate the possibilities of penance rather than the relief of guilt.

In more advanced forms of guilt, in which reactions and feelings associated with the experience have been explored, the verbal sharing of those experiences and their meaning would be helpful for the counselees. The use of authority to absolve them of responsibility may be an effective strategy with such persons. However, it should be kept in mind that individuals and couples need to be helped to verbalize the connections they have made between the problem that brings them for counseling and the imagined or real antecedent causes prior to the intervention. When this crucial step is omitted, the use of authority for absolution tends to be weakened.

Besides developmental issues, the counselees' readiness for particular strategies often needs to be taken into account in deciding which guilt-relieving tactics to employ. In this regard, the counselees generally guide the counselor, sometimes virtually verbalizing what it is they need to hear from the latter (see Example 2, below).

When the counselor's evaluation suggests that a realistic base exists for the person's guilt feelings, as it frequently does in instances involving multiple unwanted pregnancies and abortions, fetal alcohol syndrome, etc., guilt-relieving procedures may not be warranted. Rather, the counselee's feelings might be mobilized as a motivational force to assist the person to examine their behavior and to prepare for more adaptive functioning in the future.

Example 1

Guilt responses were noted in parents of a 2-year-old child with retinoblastoma. The child had one eye removed. At the time of the interview, the parents had come to the clinic for a periodic checkup for the child and for further information about the genetic disorder.[3]

1. C: I'm wondering how you feel about a decision about having kids?
2. H: Well, my decision on that is why condemn another child to having problems. . . .
3. W: [*interrupts*] I've read a lot about it. It could have been something I breathed in, that has gone wrong. . . . I could have been around you know when he was spray-painting a lot—
4. H: I get into a lot of. . . .
5. W: —a lot of really bad chemicals and I was around, remember [*to H*] in the garage, remember when you were spray-painting the boat and all the fumes and I was about 2 months pregnant . . . or not even that, I didn't realize it. Maybe I breathed in that, I don't know, you know.
6. [*C provides information regarding the early development of the eye and the probable early development of the retinoblastoma. C goes on to say:*]
7. C: So anything that happened in the second month wouldn't have affected that.
8. W: So you don't think it would really?
9. C: No, it's already past the point. . . .
10. W: Well, I wonder what could have gone wrong, I don't know.
11. C: A lot of times, we don't know. A lot of times we just have to say it was an accident and there was nothing that could have prevented it or . . . you could have stopped. That's just one thing you had no control over.
12. W: You think it could have been something in me, like I had a bad egg or something?

W presents herself as an intelligent and thinking person (3). She has given the origin of her child's problem considerable thought and has developed a seemingly plausible schema to account for it involving something external, limited, and, possibly, controllable in the future. She may harbor the hope to have more children and may be disappointed when C tells her that her explanation is based on faulty information (6). She reluctantly begins to accept internal responsibility for the child's disorder (12), but this leaves her more vulnerable and uncertain about the future.

H reveals his sense of guilt when he implies that he has experienced the affected child as a condemnation (2) a punishment—possibly for some past misdeed. He may

---

[3]The convention of rotating transcripts adopted in Kessler (1979b) will be used: C = counselor, H = husband or male partner, W = wife or female partner. Names and circumstances have been altered to maintain confidentiality.

be taking upon himself the entire responsibility for the affected child and may be bolstering his self-esteem by denying himself the pleasure of having another child and by protecting an unborn child from harm through exerting an adult level of control and responsibility.

The strategies adopted by W and H individually suggest that their separate feelings of guilt have been subjected to only a limited amount of internal processing. H appears to have dealt with his feelings by reaching a premature closure and solution. W appears to have processed her thoughts and feelings without reaching closure and thus is open to further processing following the counseling session.

C attempts to focus the couple on future reproductive considerations (1) only to discover that they have been unable to resolve their feelings of guilt over the birth of a "defective" child. The information about fetal development (7) neither addresses the couple's feelings nor the guilt–shame dynamics underlying these feelings, and this intervention has a regressive effect on W (8, 10) eventually leading to blaming herself for her misfortune (12). C's subsequent statements (11) emphasize the inability of the counselees to control events, adding to what appears to be W's growing sense of helplessness (12).

An alternative approach would have acknowledged the couple's search for an explanation, and for sense and meaning and would have shored up their need for control by emphasizing that their search is frustrated by *our* lack of knowledge and understanding of why misfortunes occur. The wording of such an intervention might be as follows: "It is quite understandable that you would be looking for some understanding as to what went wrong so that you could be comforted in knowing that you have some control in limiting future risks. But, unfortunately, *we* don't always know why these things happen. In certain aspects our knowledge is still quite inadequate and it is sad that you had to experience what we, in our ignorance, call 'accidents.'"

The acknowledgment by C that these explanations and answers are unsatisfying and that C's understanding and ability to help them is limited to reduce the couple's sense of guilt and of isolation. If the counselees continue to blame themselves, C might assure them that they are not inherently bad people and that there are limits to their levels of responsibility, that is, they can only be responsible for those events and outcomes over which they can legitimately be expected to exercise control.

Example 2

Global guilt was noted in parents of a child born with multiple congenital defects; the child died in the neonatal period. W had become pregnant while wearing an IUD and had sustained a fall early in the pregnancy. The couple waited several years before attempting the present pregnancy, which occasioned their coming for genetic counseling.

1. W: I really had bad guilt feelings, and I thought, you know, of course it was something I did, because this doesn't happen, you know, it's never happened to anyone in my family and it's, you know, it doesn't happen except to me, you know and I felt real. . . .

2. [*Further discussion of the pregnancy ensues. W then describes her interactions with the obstetrician. She says:*]

3. W: I asked him, I said, "Look, do you think that there's anything that I did that could have caused this thing?"

4. H: We never got an answer other than, "It's one in ten million."

5. [*After a brief discussion, C asks:*]

6. C: So what did you think when he told you that?

7. W: I immediately thought, the fall or the IUD or something that I did, something that I ate. I just refused to believe that it happened without a reason.

8. [*Much later in the session, the following interaction occurs:*]

9. H: It's like you're, you know, you're always looking for another answer or validation or something, probably like a detective looking for a clue.

10. C: Uh, huh.

11. W: Yeah. Why did it happen?

12. C: This thinking may go on for a period of time.

13. W: Yeah, but I think once I hear it from somebody else that. . . .

14. [*H says he accepts the rareness of the unfortunate event.*]

15 C: What do you think it was?

16. W: I think it was the IUD. I think it was the bleeding.

17. C: That's what you think?

18. W: That's what I feel. Or maybe the fall. Or maybe, smog in the city.

19. C: What do you think, Mr. A?

20. H: I think it was one in ten million, I really do.

W describes herself as having experienced guilt feelings (past tense emphasized), and it seems that no successful resolution has been reached. Her statement of self-blame (1) expresses the belief that she has taken it for granted that she has done some "wrong" and has been punished by having a child born with defects. These thoughts may be associated unconsciously with acts, thoughts, or wishes only tangentially related to the child. She appears to be experiencing a global or cosmic (Fletcher, 1972) type of guilt; of all her relatives she has been singled out for punishment. The doctor's assurance that it was a rare or freakish event (4) only exacerbated the feeling of being singled out for punishment. Her attempts to find a more direct cause (7) probably serve to protect her ego from an unknown "sin" by replacing it with a known cause that has a less condemning impact. Given the quality of her guilt experience, W is seeking forgiveness or absolution from a person in authority (13) such as the counselor or the physician. It is important to note that W has a greater preoccupation with the cause of the event than with the actual loss of the child. Thus, the reality of the loss can be dealt with adequately, but her sense of guilt remains largely unresolved.

In contrast to W, H does not seem to be disturbed by the same type of global guilt and thus is able to make use of the obstetrician's statement (4) to protect himself from self-blame.

C appears to be exploring and gathering information (6, 15, 19) and does not attempt guilt-relieving interventions. One intervention (12) incorporates a normalizing procedure but also suggests that the counselees will continue to find little relief from the nagging questions about their traumatic experience.

Given W's need for absolution, C might have used his or her authority to say something along the following lines: "You took all the necessary and normal precautions you could to promote the birth of a normal child. You followed your doctor's instructions carefully in regard to your diet, medications, exercise, and so on. What happened is *not* your fault." C might also emphasize during the course of the session that W is not a bad person, since individuals experiencing a global kind of guilt often feel that they are intrinsically bad and are to blame for the misfortunes that befall them. In such situations it may not be possible for the counselor to restructure a faulty cognitive process. However, the counselor can provide an alternate benevolent, forgiving voice, which may act as a buffer against the self-blaming tendencies.

Example 3

Iatrogenic guilt was noted in W, who has a child with a congenital heart defect.

1. [*C provides recurrence risks for congenital heart disease, emphasizing that they are low risks.*]
2. W: But, it's not a genetic thing you would say, you know, our chances are greater than anyone else who might, I mean, it's just something that could happen, right? It's nothing . . . that's a possibility. It's just something that could happen to anybody, right?
3. [*C re-emphasizes the low risks involved.*]
4. W: This is the result, like, of an aspirin or something like that. One doctor who came in said, "Nothing just happens. There's a reason for every single thing that happens. There's nothing, no such thing as just an act of nature." He said it could have been a simple aspirin at the time the heart was developing that caused it. He said it could have been something as minor as the aspirin. It could have been a cold at the time the heart was developing, that I could have been upset. . . .
5. [*C asks W how she felt about the doctor's statements.*]
6. W: That bothered me! I mean . . . you've got other kids. You don't just sit home and not get upset. You can't help not getting colds and stuff. I mean, I wasn't taking drugs or anything . . . but I did have a cold, I had the flu like in my seventh month . . . and my other child jumped on me during the third month and started some bleeding. But, I mean, that you start thinking . . . did this do that to cause this?

Here is an instance where the attempt to help the client externalize causality appears to have backfired. Blame has been inadvertently placed on W's normal, everyday (and therefore unavoidable) behaviors, that is, catching a cold, taking an aspirin, etc., events about which she ordinarily would have no reason to feel guilty. She protests that she did nothing "wrong" (6). However, a train of thought has been set in motion from which she cannot protect herself, leaving her feeling vulnerable to arbitrary and uncontrollable forces for which she has been made to feel responsible.

In her comments and questions (2) W appears willing to accept the irrationality of external causality. She seems to require a confirmation and reinforcement of that concept. C might have said, "You are perfectly right, Mrs. A. It could happen to anyone. You are not expected to be superhuman. You have to conduct your life normally to the best of your ability and that's all you or we can expect of ourselves."

Including *ourselves* in the intervention has the effect of making the interaction between the counselee and counselor an exchange between two human beings identifying with one another in their struggle to deal with one of life's major dilemmas, our inability to know in advance and control the outcome of the reproductive process.

Example 4

Developmentally advanced guilt was noted in a couple who has a 3-year-old child with a shunted hydrocephalus and who are now thinking about another pregnancy.

1. C: I wonder what it is you tell yourself about Marty's condition?
2. W: [*Among other things, she mentions that she had prolonged labor that ended with a C-section.*]
3. C: Do you think that's why Marty had the hydrocephalus?
4. W: Yes, I guess I do. Also I took aspirin during the pregnancy.
5. C: So in some ways you hold yourself responsible for the fact that Marty was born with hydrocephalus.
6. W: Yes, I know it's silly but I do.
7. C: So you know that these things had no connection with the hydrocephalus, yet on another level, you still hold yourself responsible. I wonder if you know that most couples in your situation do what you are doing, in that they wonder whether or not, if they had done something different, things would have turned out differently.
8. W: Yeah, I suppose I know but I still feel that way.
9. C: Sure, sure it does. You know there is really nothing I can say that will or can change those feelings.
10. H: At first, I blamed myself. . . . [*He goes on to describe his initial reactions and how he finally made his peace with his feelings.*]
11. C: So both of you, in your own ways, have felt some responsibility for Marty's condition.
12. W: Yes. It's better now for both of us, but every once in a while I think about it.
13. C: Uh, huh. I suppose it is difficult to accept the fact that there was nothing you might have done to change what was going to happen.

This couple appears to have been able to integrate the trauma of having had a child born with a defect and its attending guilt. W's reflective tone (8) and her appropriate self-evaluative description of the irrationality of her attributory belief (6) are indicative of an advanced level of guilt. She appears to accept her "irrational" thinking processes benignly and this makes it easy for C to agree, reinforce, and support her. Furthermore, H expresses his long struggle to come to grips with the reality of their child's problems (10). Both counselees appear to be able to differentiate between the intensity of their original reactions and their present cognitive–affective state. Presumably, the ability to integrate their experience has enabled them to contemplate the continuation of their reproductive and parenting roles.

C's interventions are nonjudgmental, empathic, and mildly probing, allowing the couple room for self-exploration and expression. By using such qualifying terms as "in some ways" (5) and "some responsibility" (11) C's interventions have a moderating tone. At the same time, they allow for the presence of some degree of irrational guilt without exaggerating its meaning or implying pathology. The couple's self-acceptance is reflected in C's comments.

Example 5

Guilt reactions were noted in the mother of an 8-month-old child who has been diagnosed as having neurofibromatosis (NF). She has brought the child, who has been developing well, to a medical genetics clinic to confirm the diagnosis. Throughout the session she never refers to the child by name, calling him "Baby" instead. On examining the child, mother, and father, the couple is informed that the diagnosis is "probable NF." The family history is unremarkable.

1. C: [*Explains the variability of the disorder, emphasizing that most cases are not severely affected and asks:*] How does that . . . sound to you?

2. W: It doesn't still sound good to me, because, uh, you know, statistically what were the chances of him getting this in the first place? Very slight. But he got it. . . . It's not reassuring . . . statistically things are kind of against us [*her voice shakes*].

3. C: It doesn't seem like you can hold out much hope right now for things to continue the way they are. . . .

4. W: [*interrupts*] Well, I, of course, I always have hope, but at two o'clock in the morning it's real hard to, uh, have hope. You kind of, you know, you just worry [*cries*]. . . .

5. C: [*Further discussion ensues after which C asks:*] How does seeing Tim [the child] functioning well and happy help you in resolving . . . [your feelings]?

6. W: That surely helps me realize that even if he has lumps that this is minor . . . What this whole thing has made me even more aware of is genetic diseases, more knowledgeable about everything, and realize how serious, really serious some cases can be, and it's kind of put me in a slump, not just for my own predicament, but for the predicament of other mothers. . . .

7. C: You're a lot more sensitive to what a lot of people go through or take for granted.

8. W: Right, and, uh, you know, I never took it for granted that this wasn't going to happen to me. I never considered a genetic disease, but I was so concerned about how I took care of myself when I was pregnant, overly, in fact. People would even say I was even a little fanatic about not wearing nail polish and not cleaning my oven and not painting anything, not eating, drinking, or doing anything that, I've always been, didn't want to take any unnecessary chances and to have this thrown at me, this is really uh [*she breaks off*] not ever. . . .

9. C: This is something you had no control over.

10. W: No and, uh, I had never read, ever about a new mutation for a genetic disease. If I had even suspected if we had even the slightest thought a genetic disease was in our family, I just would have adopted a baby. I never would have taken a chance on having a baby, ever. But it's . . . [*cries*].

W appears to be unreasurred and inconsolable (2, 4) despite C's attempts (1, 5) to emphasize the positive side of things. Her reactions display an element of narcissistic injury (6, 8) and her thinking indicates an obsessional intrusion of calamitous ideas (2, 4, 6). Her sense of guilt appears to be unconscious and this is evident in the use of the double negative (8). She appears to have taken it for granted that her child would be born with a defect and she graphically describes (8) her near compulsive attempts at warding off punishment. It is unclear why she was so concerned; presumably she felt guilt about something even prior to the actual birth or pregnancy. It is conceivable that her defensive precautions (8) may have the effect of absolving her from some of the responsibility for the disorder. After all, didn't she take every possible precaution to protect the fetus from harm? Unconsciously, she may have been ambivalent about having this child (10, and the fact that she does not use the child's name).

W's guilt feelings appear to have remained largely unchanged since the child's birth, presumably because of their unconscious nature. In deciding on specific interventions, C would need to ascertain the degree to which W's guilt feelings are adversely affecting her parenting, thoughts about further reproductive decisions, present mental health, etc.

C's comments do not appear to be as effective as they might be. C tries to minimize the child's disorder (1), presumably to relieve W's fears and concerns. When W expresses her lack of reassurance, C attempts to interpret (3) W's negativity. W seems to hear the interpretation as a personal criticism and responds defensively (4). C then attempts (5) to lead W to realize that things are not as bad as she believes they are. This also seems to be nonproductive (6). C does not appear to be taking W's defensiveness and psychological needs into account in his or her statements. Thus, C's efforts to help W achieve insight into her own behavior—an approach that might be effective if C had an unlimited amount of time and multiple subsequent sessions—does not appear to be working. In our opinion, C may need to have played a more active role in shaping W's cognitive processes along more self-enhancing and adaptive paths. For example, C might have responded to W's lack of reassurance (2) with a statement affirming that it is understandable that she would be doubtful and concerned about statistical odds of things, but that the reality is that she must be doing "good" as a mother because her child is developing so well. Also, rather than emphasizing W's lack of control over events (9), C might have emphasized how sensitive and caring a person W was to have made such enormous efforts and how indicative this was of the fact that she is basically a good and loving person. These interventions would be directed toward W's guilt feelings and toward bolstering her self-esteem and maternal self-image.

SHAME-REDUCING TACTICS

Dynamically, persons experiencing shame are fearful that if they expose their "shame," others will not think well of them or they will be subject to scorn, ridicule, and rejection. Exposure and confession are thus filled with considerable anxiety and fear. Therefore, it is imperative that the counselor remains nonjudgmental. The relief that comes after the person has "confessed" and has not had their worst fears confirmed is sometimes visibly noticeable. Even when it is not noticeable, confession generally results in giving people a virtual "new lease on life," freeing them to devote their attention and energies to other important tasks.

Tactics in dealing with shame responses include:

Developing a working alliance. The counselees need to believe that the counselor is on their side, will not be judgmental, and will work actively to promote their interests.

Evoking feelings. The counselor needs to help the counselees to express their feelings and to respond empathetically. In general, there is a salutary effect resulting from interactions in which counselees expose their shame and the counselor responds with nonjudgmental acceptance.

Accentuating the positive. The counselor should point out and accentuate areas of functioning where counselees are doing well. When self-esteem is down, the person tends to be blind to possibilities that they may actually be making the right decisions and be functioning effectively.

Ego-bolstering. The counselor needs to be rewarding, emphasizing how good the counselees are as people or parents, how clever they may be for finding such-and-such solutions to their problems, and other ego-enhancing tactics.

Where more intense (less well-articulated) forms of shame are present, the primary counseling task is to develop an alliance with the counselees. The counselor needs to be accepting and nonjudgmental. This necessitates that he or she be aware of possible negative or judgmental feelings toward the counselees that the latter may have evoked. Awareness of such reactions is the first step in preventing inadvertently negative and inappropriate remarks from impeding the counselor's effectiveness. In developing an alliance with the counselees, the counselor needs to encourage actively the former to recognize or to label their emotional experience—shame—and help them see that their feelings are dictating their behavior. In addition, the counselees may need to be encouraged to try out new behaviors. Once a working alliance is formed with the counselees, the counselor might do well to be directive in reshaping their behavior in more adaptive and productive directions. One means of achieving this end is to utilize paradoxical interventions. For example, if the counselor is dealing with a couple who is hiding their child away and thus limiting the child's social contact with peers, he or she might say something along the following lines: "I know you are doing the best for your child, and your child needs contact with other children. Let's see how we can find ways to help meet your child's needs for social contact."

By emphasizing that the counselees are doing the best they can (even though this may be nonproductive or ineffective) the counselor accomplishes two things. It helps him or her be more empathic to the counselee's situation; indeed, they are doing their best. Second, it gives the counselees a message that bolsters their self-esteem because their efforts are being recognized as positive rather than as negative ones. Without saying to them that their efforts are useless or worthless (and hence, that they [the counselees] are worthless), the counselor points out the possibility of alternate and perhaps more effective ways of coping with the child's situation. Opening up this spectrum of possibilities may lead to an increase in the counselee' s self-esteem, for now they may be able to see that there is something (else) that can be done about the problems they face.

Example 6

Advanced shame reactions were noted in a father of a child with Apert syndrome.

1. H: My wife copes with it . . . better than I do. I keep . . . to myself most the time . . . At first a newborn with some type of deformity or something wrong you're not real sure what they're going to be able to accomplish and you think . . . I'm . . . going to be here the rest of my life with some vegetable. She's [the child] obviously not a vegetable and it's like now she's doing all these cute and encouraging things and that's helped us get over all of our fears more than all the doctors and the books and everything. . . .

2. C: You said that your wife is able to talk a lot more about Mary. Who is she able to talk to?

3. H: Ah, well her friends. It's like she's real up front and she'll be out shopping . . . and people will say to her. "Oh what a cute baby!" And then they'll see her hands and then they'll say, "Oh, what's wrong with her?" And she goes, "Oh, she's got Apert's syndrome . . ." and just goes on. It just runs off like water off a duck. But, to me, it's sort of, I'm not embarrassed, but I try to avoid people if I can and I don't try to get into talks about her [the child's] problems, unless I have to. . . .

4. C: What makes you want to avoid it?

5. H: Oh, I guess psychologically I sort of feel responsible in a way. It is sort of like if there's something wrong with your kid there's something wrong with you. I don't know, it's some really weird little head trip I really shouldn't have but it's just sort of there.

6. C: [*Discusses dominant inheritance and then says:*] You said that you don't like to talk about the fact that Mary has Apert's syndrome. But, when you have talked about it, has it helped at all?

7. H: I can't . . . I try to avoid it now. All my friends . . . encourage me that it's nothing you did or it's not your fault. But, okay but I'm not embarrassed. It's a hard adjective. I don't even know what the adjective is, but it's frustrating and tired and it's a hard one to explain. This would be a great one for a psychiatrist's office . . . Well, I'm not sure if it helps or not. I want to avoid it . . . I don't know. So it's hard.

8. H: [*He talks briefly about his frustrations and continues:*]

9. H: It's like they [others] say, "What caused it?" Well, I don't know. "Well, can it be fixed?" Well, I don't know. "Well, can they fix her hands?" Well, the state of the art is improving, so I don't know. So, it's hard.

10. H: [*He goes on to reveal that he is anticipating that Mary will be teased by other children and he is already planning to teach her martial arts so that she can be tough and defend herself. He goes on to say:*]

11. H: I feel bad, but it's not this overpowering thing that weighs down my mind all the time like this real heavy depression. It's just those isolated times, like once a week or something when you feel shy, standoffish and protective, like I don't want you in my space, man, you know, just leave my baby alone, you know—

12. C: Uh huh.

13. H: —and, I find myself when I know I'm going shopping . . . We've got two baby girls, I've got my choice. I can take this one or this one. If I'm not going someplace where I'm going to be in public, I find myself not taking Mary. I'll take Ann [the unaffected daughter]. But, if I'm going to the beach to sit in the sun or something, I'll take Mary with me. I noticed that when I have my choices and it's going to be a crowded situation, I choose the one that looks normal, you know, with people I don't know. I'll take Mary, which is kind of unfair too, but I have noticed that . . . it's not fair, but I make it up to her by, she gets to go on the beach. Okay, like I don't take her to the supermarket . . . but I take her to the beach. She'd rather go to the beach anyway, but it's in my head why she doesn't go to the supermarket. [It's] not because it's not her turn. . . .

14. [*After some discussion, H says:*]

15. H: I'm not ashamed, don't get me wrong. And, I'm not ashamed of myself. But, there's still this weird adjective, I don't know what . . . it is. . . .

H is very articulate and self-revealing; his sense of shame permeates this entire transcript. One can also sense his affection for the child and his ability to form a genuine attachment to her. His shame is more of himself, and his own inadequacy and inability to produce a normal child than it is of the child. Therefore, one finds the affection for the child coupled with his personal sense of shame. H, therefore, can relate to the child in private situations but has difficulty in the public arena (13).

It is easy to confuse shame and guilt in his sense of responsibility for the child's condition (5) but his feeling that there is something wrong with the child and, therefore, by extension, with himself rather than with something that he did, is the trademark of the shame state. Despite his assertion (3, 7) that he is not embarrassed (by which he means he does not redden), H's defensive posture of avoidance (3, 7), hiding (13), and withdrawal (3) all indicate shame. In this case, the defensive behavior has become a fixed part of his responses and is no longer a transient response, like embarrassment. The defensive behavior may serve to protect him from an awareness of his feelings, so that he is only aware of a "weird" unidentifiable feeling (7, 15). His confusion and concern about his feelings and behavior and his offhand reference to the psychiatrist's office (7) may indicate a request for permission to obtain psychological assistance.

C's approach appears to be effective in helping H talk about his feelings and concerns. In do doing C has uncovered areas of H's present and future parenting that may be (or become) maladaptive (10, 13). C might have dealt with these issues by making some positive comments about his affection for Mary, his wish not to discriminate between his two daughters, and his continued personal suffering because this "weird" feeling is interfering with his ability to live up to his own standard of parenting. Also, C might go on to emphasize that H might want to avail himself of counseling in order to discover what it is that is interfering with such admirable wishes. In other words, H may need to seek help in order to overcome his personal handicaps and to further his fathering capacity.

Example 7: The Shame Couple

C.C., a well-educated 35-year-old woman, was referred for preamniocentesis counseling by her obstetrician because of maternal age. She and her husband came to the counseling session confused and enraged at both her physician and the genetic counselor, whom they had just met. The couple has two normal children and C.C. strongly asserted that these pregnancies were uncomplicated and that their two children were healthy and beautiful. The current pregnancy was desired and she and her husband were overjoyed at its confirmation. When their physician made the referral, the joy turned to sadness and rage. They felt singled out and stigmatized. They said that they had never heard of amniocentesis and upon being referred they immediately felt that there must be something wrong with them or their fetus. She repeatedly questioned the counselor as to why she hadn't been referred with her previous pregnancy 2 years earlier. "What was so different now?" When C attempted to provide the couple with data on the general risk for birth defects in any pregnancy, they were particularly disturbed because they had not acknowledged or entertained the possibility, either then or previously, that they might have a child with a defect. The couple had considerable difficulty deciding whether or not to have the amniocentesis procedure.

This is an example of less advanced shame in a couple apparently vulnerable to narcissistic injuries. The rage expressed at the counselor was a response to the threat of possibly being exposed as being less than perfect. One can easily imagine that the counselor might be caught by surprise by the intensity of their rage and thus respond defensively in this kind of situation. No injury had actually occurred. A service had merely been offered with the intention of preventing future injuries. Why the rage? We suggest that for this couple the sense of losing control coupled with the slightest suspicion of imperfection and a vulnerability to narcissistic injury are sufficient to evoke strong defensive reactions: self-esteem appears to be fragile and cannot tolerate any degree of exposure. C might feel wrongly attacked and, therefore, is primed to respond in an overt or covert aggressive or emotionally distancing manner. C might protect himself or herself by realizing that the couple's rage is not a personal attack but rather an expression of a deeply felt fear of exposure of one's inadequacies. Understanding and empathizing with their anxiety should help the counselor to maintain an appropriate counseling distance.

C's major counseling task is to develop a working relationship with the counselees, help them obtain a sense of control, and allow them to behave in a more mature fashion. Their sense of outrage and the feeling that they have been attacked may need to be assuaged while simultaneously challenging them to behave in a mature and responsible fashion. A paradoxical intervention may be helpful in this regard. C might agree with the couple that they are, indeed, very responsible and competent people, and, as such, would surely want to be aware of the latest medical advances and technologies so that they could continue to be the excellent parents that they are. Given their good reproductive history (i.e., their negative family history of genetically related problems) and the reality of their age-appropriate risk for a chromosomal disorder, they would have a relatively small chance of producing a defective child, but would they want to take that or any risk?

Raging or rageful clients and patients are among the most difficult ones with whom professionals need to deal. They tend to evoke anger and rejection among helping professionals and their expectations of rejection, poor service, and disappointment is frequently self-fulfilling. When the professional can establish a working alliance and provide empathy to them, such persons can swiftly switch to a delightfully cooperative and pleasing way of functioning.

Example 8

A mixture of guilt and shame were noted in a mother of a child with a congenital malformation. The mother had recently undergone a therapeutic abortion, one of several over the past 5 years since the child's birth.

1. W: I feel like a murderer . . . I really do [*cries*]. What can I say, it's not like you've had a miscarriage. That's not your fault. But, you know, I guess it's my

family background. I've always been raised religiously and everything. I feel like, in God's eyes, he really looks down on me, and, it's not just God, myself.

2. C: It sounds to me that you're disappointed in what you've done.

3. W: You should have heard the expressions in their [the doctors] voices when I told them I had those abortions. . . .

4. C: I can see how much this hurts you and I can see how harshly you've already judged yourself. It seems to me that as you look back at the decisions you've made, they haven't made you feel very good about yourself. I'm wondering what thoughts you've given to steps that would prevent that from happening again?

W is clearly expressing feelings of guilt (1), and since it is of a total, global, and unredeeming nature, it is an example of a less advanced form of guilt. Her guilt also appears to have strong overtones of shame as expressed in her image of God looking down on her and the feelings of reproach and shame in His eyes. Because she identifies with God as an ego ideal, she too looks down on and condemns herself. She is responding to the willfulness of her acts as opposed to the chance happening of a miscarriage which could have absolved her of the responsibility of having to make a personal decision. C does not attempt to alleviate her guilt feelings (2) and the focus of the later intervention (4) is on helping W find more adaptive responses, ones that would lead to a greater control over events and a raising of her self-esteem.

Example 9

Intense shame and defensive guilt were noted in a 41-year-old mother of a child born 4 years earlier with trisomy 18. She had recently become pregnant and had been referred for genetic counseling by a nurse practitioner. Her husband was not enthusiastic about the referral and did not come to the session. Just before the appointment, she miscarried, much to her relief.

1. W: We've gone through the whole family history. There is absolutely nothing on either side of the family . . . which, of course, dumps the guilt back on me. I then go back to the same thing, what did I do wrong?

2. C: Uh huh. Did you ever consider the possibility that you did nothing wrong?

3. W: Yes, but I also come back to thinking, what did I do wrong? See, I can't resolve that. There's no way to go back in time.

4. C: Right. And there's no way of changing what happened.

5. W: So, uh, I kind of have to put that out of the way and say, "Here's today, and tomorrow. What am I going to do tomorrow?" Uh, there are things I would do differently, uh, I think the stress factor [*pause*] had some bearing on it.

6. [*Further discussion ensues in which she describes her relationship with her husband. This is her second marriage and she has a normal child from her*

first marriage. The birth of the child with the chromosome disorder led to a brief separation from the present husband and continuing marital difficulties. She was severely depressed following the child's birth and subsequent death. C takes a family history during the course of which the following exchange occurs:]

7. W: I'm the problem. . . .

8. C: You're only one person in the family—

9. W: [*interrupts*] In the entire family—

10. C: —to have a child with problems?

11. W: —with problems. So, which would make me wonder what went wrong?

12. C: Have you talked about this with your family at all?

13. W: Oh, you can't talk to my family. Oh my God, this is, this was a disaster in my family . . . Nobody wanted to deal with it, so I decided I'd try to deal with it myself [*nervous laugh*].

14. C: And what did H tell his family?

15. W: Oh, . . . they got copies of the medical reports. I didn't find this necessary at all.

16. C: How did they get copies of the medical reports?

17. W: Well [he] got his whole family involved in this thing. On top of all my grief and everything, I had to deal with his family.

18. C: How did you feel about them knowing?

19. W: I felt terrible. I didn't feel that this was the way it should've been handled at all. And so it was just compounding my grief.

20. C: And so you weren't talking to his family?

21. W: Oh, he wanted to sue people, this man, he was so irrational . . . He just got so excited, and you couldn't talk to him.

22. [*Pregnancy history is obtained. C asks W if the child had been named and she replies, "David." C continues:*]

23. C: When you think of your son, do you think of him as David?

24. W: No, I don't associate that name with him at all.

25. C: Why do you think that is?

26. W: [*pause*] Uh, I, I, uh, I don't accept it . . . I don't accept the baby.

27. C: How do you not accept him?

28. W: As being real. As being a real person.

29. C: How much did you get a chance to look at him?

30. W: I saw him for 10 seconds. I never saw him again . . . I saw a very deformed child that looked like a baby, but wasn't a baby. The eyes were just vacant.

31. [*After a brief exchange, C inquires whether W had asked where the child was taken.*]

32. W: I didn't really talk to anybody. I just stayed in my room . . . after he was born, I was . . . brought into a room [*pause*] and I was in there with other women, who whispered quite a bit to themselves, and they decided to move me to another room, and I knew something was wrong and I said I wanted to see the baby . . . And they brought him, and I looked at him and I couldn't look at him again.

33. C: What were you feeling then?

34. W: Horror. Absolute horror.

35. C: Horror that. . . .

36. W: Horror that he could look like that, be born like that . . . Everything was wrong. Everything was in the wrong place. Everything connected up wrong . . . I could never describe the feeling. I don't think that unless you've experienced it, you could ever understand.

37. C: Can you give me some idea what it was like?

38. W: Just a sense of absolute hopelessness, and despair. Uh [*begins to cry*], hopelessness. Can't change anything. . . .

39. C: That's right.

40. W: Can't change the fact [*pause; sighs; stops crying*]. I cried so much I swore I would never cry again. And I didn't cry for a long, long time. I cried and cried. I'd cry in the car, I'd cry if anyone looked at me the wrong way, I spent a whole year crying. And then I decided I wouldn't cry ever again [*pause*]. And I didn't. I wouldn't cry at anything for a long, long time.

W's sense of guilt is apparent from the onset (1, 3, 5, 11). It is largely unresolved and apparently unintegrated (3). The guilt is global (7, 9, 11), it lacks self-forgiveness (3), and W does not appear to have found a cognitive framework in which her traumatic experiences can be given meaning (40). The peremptory rejection (3) of C's attempt to relieve the guilt (2) suggests that these feelings may subserve important defensive functions (see below).

Evidence for intense feelings of shame emerge slowly over the course of the session (13, 26, 36, 38) and are especially prominent as C encourages W to talk about her experience with the child. W describes feelings of isolation (13, 26, 32, withdrawal (32), wanting to hide her eyes (32), helplessness (38), and, above all, the rejection of her child as being a part of herself (24, 26, 30), and the horror of the shame (34) of having produced such a monstrous thing (36). In rejecting the child, W has probably made it difficult, if not impossible, to find an adequate emotional resolution of her feelings. Presumably, this has left her in a state of shame. However, the feelings of shame do not appear to be experienced because her attention is focused on the less distressing feelings of guilt (1).

W's description of H's response to the birth of their child (21) is one associated with the rage of the narcissistically injured individual. In turn, W's apparently unresolved anger toward H (21) suggest that their earlier marital difficulties (6) have not been resolved entirely. Given a certain amount of self-centeredness and a lack of empathy for H (17, 19) and his apparent lack of support and empathy for her, W has probably had to withdraw emotionally (40) and has not been able to integrate the experience on her own.

C's interventions have encouraged W to "tell her story" and to express her emotions. Noteworthy is C's simple, accepting, empathic statement (37) that allows W to experience the intensity of her feelings about the events of the past and finally permits her to cry. Having opened herself emotionally, W now is in need of help and guidance to begin the process of cognitive restructuring and to find meaning in her experiences. Several examples of potential interventions follow:

- Dealing with W's sense of guilt (1, 3) and her need to put these feelings behind her (5) and, possibly, make amends, C might have inquired what specifically she might do differently if she had another opportunity.
- When W says that she is the only one in her family with problems (7, 11), C might have attempted a normalizing tactic such as, "It is understandable that when no one else in your family has a problem, you would wonder why this has happened to me and, like most anyone else, you would try to make some sense out of it. One way a lot of people make sense out of the problems they have is to blame themselves. It sometimes feels better to blame yourself than to think things like this happen by chance or for no reason."
- In response to W's tears (38) C might have provided a summary statement along the lines of, "Whatever else the current pregnancy and miscarriage has meant to you, it has given you a chance to look at the painful experiences of the past from the vantage point of today. Sometimes all one can do about some of the scars of the past is to cry, and both you and your husband have your share of scars to cry about. Perhaps now is the time to also give some thought to how the two of you can heal the still-open wounds that may exist so that you find the solace and comfort you obviously deserve." C might then deal with W's reproductive (or contraceptive) plans, explore the need or desire for marital or individual therapy, and provide her with encouragement that although she has been hurt in the past, she has good years ahead that need to be lived as best she can.

ACKNOWLEDGMENTS

We thank Mr. Toney Pennewell for typing this manuscript.

REFERENCES

Erikson EH (1963) Childhood and Society. New York: WW Norton.

Fletcher J (1972) The brink: the parent-child bond in the genetic revolution. Theol Stud 33:457–485.

Harvey J, Smith W (1977) Social Psychology: An Attributional Approach. St. Louis: CV Mosby Co.

Hecht F, Holmes LB (1972) What we don't know about genetic counseling. New Engl J Med 287:464–465.

Hsia YS (1979) The genetic counselor as information giver. Birth Defects: Original Article Series 15:169–186.

Jones, E, Davis V, Gergen K (1961) Role playing variations and their informational value for person perception. J Abnorm Soc Psychol 63:302–310.

Kessler S (1979a) The psychological foundations of genetic counseling. In: Kessler S (ed). Genetic Counseling: Psychological Dimensions. New York: Academic Press, pp 17–33.

Kessler S (1979b) The genetic counseling session. In: Kessler S (ed). Genetic Counseling: Psychological Dimensions. New York: Academic Press, pp 65–105.

Kohlberg L (1963) Moral development and identification. In: Stevenson H (ed). Child Psychology. Chicago: University of Chicago Press, pp. 277–332.

Kohut H (1971) The Analysis of Self. New York: International Universities Press.

Lewis HB (1971) Shame and Guilt in Neurosis. New York: International Universities Press.

Lynd HM (1958) On Shame and the Search for Identity. New York: Harcourt Brace, and World, Inc.

Piaget J (1948) The Moral Judgment of the Child. New York: Free Press.

Piers G, Singer MB (1953) Shame and Guilt. Springfield, IL: CC Thomas.

Ruma EH, Mosher DL (1967) Relationship between moral judgment and guilt in delinquent boys. J Abnorm Psychol 72:122–127.

Targum SD (1981) Psychotherapeutic considerations in genetic counseling. Am J Med Genet 8:281–289.

4

Suffering and Countertransference[1]

As part of a recent conference dealing with the general topic of difficult situations for genetic counselors I had an opportunity to pull together some thoughts about the issue of countertransference that I would like to expand on here. At the conference, three genetic counselors shared their personal experiences dealing with problems that counselees often have, but in this case the shoe was on the other foot. Not only did the counselors have to deal with difficulties in their own lives but they all continued to work and deal with counselees who had similar and, at times, the same problem they had to face. When the discussion was opened to the audience, other poignant stories emerged and, all in all, the participants and many in the audience left deeply touched by the struggles of our colleagues as well as by those of our counselees.

As professionals, we need to integrate our external professional lives with our inner experiences (and vice versa). Thus we need to acknowledge that no one is immune to pain and suffering. The laws of chance operate for genetic counselors just as they do for everyone else. "Bad" things do happen to genetic counselors. But even if they do not, we are as vulnerable as the next person to experience loss and pain. Disappointment, loss, feelings of being rejected and misunderstood, of failure, embarrassment, hurt, and so on are ubiquitous human phenomena. No one is exempt.

When counselors experience the same kind of problems their clients are dealing with, or problems sufficiently similar to their own, it inevitably affects them as individuals and it changes the character of their work. It does so in many ways. Some counselors report that they became more patient with clients, but others found themselves being more impatient. Almost all had to struggle with the problem of

[1]This essay first appeared as Kessler S (1992) Psychological aspects of genetic counseling. VIII. Suffering and countertransference. *Journal of Genetic Counseling* 1:303–308. Reprinted with kind permission of the publisher, Kluwer Academic/Human Sciences Press.

containment of feelings and of at least two kinds of countertransferential reactions, associative and projective.

Clients' experiences provoke our own associations, thoughts, and images. For example, the former may be sharing with you some benign thoughts about gardening and the pretty flowers that she picked yesterday. As the counselor listens, images of flowers may flash across the inner mental screen and unbidden feelings of sadness and loss may arise as the counselor remembers the child she might have had (or the one that was stillborn) whom she was planning to name Daisy. Such associations may lead to others and before the counselor knows it she may no longer be attending to what the counselee is saying and feeling but to her own internal voice and suffering. Even if the counselor is (partially) attending, these associations may impede or interfere with the total understanding of the counselee.

Not all of our associations will be to things happening in our contemporary lives or in the recent past. Many of our associations may be (perhaps subliminal) memories of things that we experienced as children or young adults, which become active in our minds as we listen to and try to understand our counselees' experiences. Thus, on one level, these associations assist us to provide empathy and understanding. On the other hand, these associations remind us of our own losses and traumas.

Over and over again in counseling and psychotherapy, professionals are continually exposed to material that tends to re-open their own past and current wounds, reminding them of their personal inadequacies, failures, losses, and the like. As professionals, our ability to resolve past hurt is constantly being challenged. When loss is fresh in memory, the "wounds" are still open and reminders from our clients tend to keep them open. This becomes particularly problematic when the counselor's personal pain, whether to current or past losses and traumas, leads him or her to begin to identify with the client through projection. Also, if the counselor's own habitual way of dealing with internal pain and past wounds is through emotional distancing, then these constant reminders tend to interfere with this psychological strategy and lead either to a "hardening" of the defenses or to a need to reappraise and confront personal wounds. The former consequence may render the counselor "useless" from the counselee's perspective since the counselor is liable to lose altogether his or her ability to be empathic. The latter strategy, although involved with greater distress and angst, has greater promise for personal growth.

Another situation in which the counselors' associations may lead to countertransferential difficulties occurs when they assume that they understand one counselee based on the experiences dealing with the same or similar problem in another counselee. The inferences drawn from the previous experiences become applied to a current situation, sometimes without fully taking into account the subtle differences between the cases (and invariably there are always subtle differences in family dynamics, life history, etc.). This often results in attempts to provide empathy that may not even be appropriate for the situation.

Projective identification with the client is another form of countertransference. In this case, the identification often leads to some understanding of the client's inner world. Because the counselor has suffered, he or she "understands" the client's suffering. For example, because a counselor may have had a therapeutic abortion following the identification of a fetus with a chromosomal abnormality, she is in position to understand how a woman facing the same problem might be dealing with it and might be feeling. However, there is another side to projective identification. For example, one's own pain may become so acute that we might counsel the client to distance themselves from their problem in order to reduce our own inner distress. We often do so in the guise of helping the client focus their attention on less distressing thoughts, feelings, and images. In other words, we lose our sense of whose discomfort is being managed in our intervention, the client's or our own. We have projected our thoughts and feelings and made them the client's.

Projective identification with the client gives the professional the sense that they understand the client and because they do that they can be empathic. But this may be misleading. Cassel (1991) and others point out that we can never really know or understand another's suffering. Thus, counselors often make the mistake of thinking that because they have had a problem similar to that of their client they *ipso facto* understand and have empathy for the other. Often the empathy is shallow because the projective identification, if expressed, frequently leads to premature closure in an interchange with a client. The inquiry about the counselee's perceptions, thoughts, and feelings becomes truncated. For example, imagine a situation in which your child comes home crying, and you ask him what the matter is, and he tells you that his friend next door doesn't want to play with him. You identify with him because it is likely that something similar has happened to you when you were a child. You experience the upset and hurt you experienced back, then projecting these feelings on the child. You comfort the child's hurt and perhaps say to him that children sometimes can be silly and fickle and you send him to play alone. Now imagine a second version of the same scenario. Your child comes home crying, and you inquire what the matter is, and the child says the same thing. As in the first scenario, you remember your own hurt as a child when this happened to you, however, you contain your own pain and ask the child if the friend had told him why he doesn't want to play with him (notice how the inquiry is being expanded). Imagine now the child replies that his friend's parent told his friend not to play with your child (new information). This might intensify your own identification with the child because again this was a hurt you also experienced and you might be tempted to project these feelings on the child. Nevertheless, again you contain your own feelings and hurt and you make further inquiry and you learn that his friend's parent does not approve of your family or of your family's ethnicity or religion and thus does not want his child to play with yours. Again there is an opportunity to projectively identify with your child and again you contain your feelings and say to your child something to the effect that not only can you understand why your child is unhappy but you can also understand that his friend may be unhappy about the situation too.

In the example above, notice how different the level of understanding and empathy is in the two instances. Note in the first scenario that the inquiry of the child is curtailed so that important facts that change the meaning of the child's experience fail to emerge. This does not mean that the parent was not empathic toward the child, but the empathy was not very deep. Note also what it is the child learns in the two situations about friendship and about the availability of the parent for comforting and for making sense out of a seemingly senseless situation.

Analogous situations frequently occur in the counseling encounter. Counselors and psychotherapists struggle constantly with the issue of projective identification and those who master and contain their projections tend to provide deeper levels of empathy than those who do not. One of the major pitfalls in the counseling profession and a problem all counselors share is the tendency to delude ourselves that we understand the other person. Often we do not.

One of the issues that emerged in the conference was the degree to which counselors should share their personal experiences with their clients. One side of the problem is that some clients ask their counselors whether or not the latter have had children, an amniocentesis, abortion, abnormal results, etc., and some counselors frankly said they felt inadequate if they had not had these experiences and did not know how to handle the situation. The degree of defensiveness on the part of some counselors raises concerns about the quality of counseling training genetic counseling programs provide them; this is an issue that students should be comfortable with before they graduate as counselors. On the other hand, counselors who have had adverse experiences were tempted to tell their clients about it, especially when challenged by clients who received "bad" news and implied that counselors did or would not understand them. Several counselors reported that when their clients were in an inconsolable rage about the news they received they tended to inform them about their own experience to provide them with understanding (empathy) as well as some perspective. This seemed to have a calming effect on some clients. However, one of the participants said that this strategy did not always work for her.

I had, and continue to have, reservations about disclosing aspects of one's personal life in the counseling context, mostly because the perceived calming effect on the client may be the result of an arousal of concern for the counselor's emotional state. Thus, the client may end up taking care of the counselor rather than focusing on their own suffering. This may be productive for some clients, at least in the short run. However, counselors should be sure that this strategy does not have the more unconscious need to defuse the inconsolable ragings of the client so that we obtain greater comfort. After all, raging clients are often difficult to deal with even in the best of circumstances. It would be important for counselors to follow up clients with whom they have shared their painful life experiences to determine the longer range impact of such interventions.

In general, I take a dim view of sharing with clients details of one's own personal life. Genetic counselors, still insecure in their professional role, often tend to share (inappropriately) pieces of information about themselves, such as their home telephone numbers, in an attempt to "buy" acceptance and friendship. I have heard all sorts of rationalizations for such practices, but am still unconvinced that they either help the client or lead to a maturation of professionalism for the counselor. In fact, such practices often lead to boundary problems with some clients that tend to repeat similar conflicts they have experienced in the past. Clients need to obtain friendship from others, not from counselors who have a very different role to play with them. Part of this role is being friendly to the counselee but not being their friend, and there is a major difference between the two phenomena. On their side, counselors also need to find friendship and sources of self-worth from persons other than their clients.

Another situation that tended to evoke one's own personal suffering or counter-transferential responses is that of couples seeking sex selection. Counselors at the conference often felt (and sometimes expressed) outrage at the contrast between their own difficulty in achieving reproductive "success" and what they saw as either a "wasteful" or frivolous use of genetic technology. There was also a sense of sadness about the thought that some people had the wherewithal to conceive and produce a healthy child and squandered that opportunity.

Sex selection appears to be one of those issues that evokes enormous emotion in counselors (and others) and almost always leads to countertransferential problems. It seems that the profession as a whole needs to take a deeper look at the issues raised by this topic and devote time at national meetings to exploring its meaning, counseling strategies that seem to work, suggested institutional changes, and so on. A provocative discussion of some of the ethical issues raised by sex selection may be found in Wertz and Fletcher (1989).

Considering the extent to which countertransference is evoked in the context of genetic counseling (Kessler, 1979), greater attention needs to be paid to it. The responsible counselor has an obligation to be aware of countertransferential potentiality and, if necessary, to seek out and obtain professional assistance in dealing with clients who evoke such responses. The initial step in dealing with countertransference is to recognize it when it occurs and to see it for what it is. The fact that genetic counselors are now discussing these issues in a public forum attests to their awareness of these issues and their growing professional maturity.

REFERENCES

Cassel FJ (1991) Recognizing suffering. Hastings Center Rep 21(3):24–31.

Kessler S (1979) The genetic counselor as psychotherapist. Birth Defects: Original Article Series 15(2):187–200.

Wertz DC, Fletcher JC (1989) Fatal knowledge? Prenatal diagnosis and sex selection. Hastings Center Rep 19(3):21–27.

5

Preselection: A Family Coping Strategy in Huntington Disease[1]

INTRODUCTION

One of the major contributions of genetics to human welfare is the reduction of reproductive uncertainty. Thus, a pregnant woman who undergoes amniocentesis is reassured that she does not carry a fetus with Down syndrome, a condition unwanted by prospective parents. However, in many genetic disorders, multiple uncertainties continue to exist. For some, like Huntington disease (HD), the delayed age of onset and the impossibility (until recently) of determining in advance who will be affected exact an enormous psychological toll (Wexler, 1979). In such instances, denial or magical thinking often are major strategies of coping; "patient preselection" is one example. In this paper, the preselection phenomenon will be considered, particularly in relation to HD, although it is often observed in other situations involving genetic or late-onset diseases (e.g., Alzheimer's disease).

THE PRESELECTION PHENOMENON

Preselection is a family system phenomenon. Preselection refers to the singling out, in advance, of an asymptomatic relative to become eventually the "affected" individual. This preselection often involves a child and, in the case of HD, generally occurs when the parent first begins to show symptoms. The "sick" role is assigned to a relative, and the behavior of the individual relatives tends to be organized around beliefs

[1]This essay first appeared as Kessler S (1988) Invited essay on the psychological aspects of genetic counseling. V. Preselection: a family coping strategy in Huntington disease. *American Journal of Medical Genetics* 31:617–621. Reprinted with kind permission of the publisher, John Wiley and Sons.

consistent with such assignment. By preselecting a potential patient, the family creates the illusion that a reduction has been achieved in the multiple uncertainties inherent in the disorder, that is, its genetic transmission, its delayed age of onset, and the uncertain status of the individual at risk. It is as if the chance nature of gene transmission is brought under control and the chronic threat of stochastic processes has been defused.

The process of preselection is unconscious on the part of the relatives, and preselected individuals are generally unaware of their central psychological role in the family. Once preselection occurs, the choice is supported and reinforced by repeated association with the affected parent or the parent's family. The processes of identification are used to support the myth that the individual will eventually be affected by HD. Behavior linking the person to the affected parent is highlighted and the perception reinforced—"That's what Mom used to do"; "Dad walked that way"—so that the preselected persons and the other relatives come to believe that their created scenario is the only one possible.

MECHANISMS OF PRESELECTION

Naming a child after the affected parent may be a step toward the later preselection of that individual as a potentially affected individual. In one case, a couple had three children, the youngest of whom was named after the father, who subsequently developed HD. Soon after the diagnosis was made, the wife divorced her husband, took custody of the children, and several years later remarried. By the time the youngest child began school, he was identified as having behavior difficulties at home and in school. He was diagnosed as hyperactive and was treated with Ritalin for a short period of time. By his mother's report, he had a learning disability and a history of frequent truancy. She described him as being "impossible to live with" from an early age and as being "just like his father," whereas the older children were held out as models of perfection. He was unable to accept his new stepfather, and there were repeated conflicts and arguments with his mother, generally ending with his being punished or running away from home. By age 15 years, he was brought to a psychiatrist, who placed him in a locked facility and prescribed neuroleptics.

In another family in which the father was affected with HD, the two children had quite different perceptions of their childhood. One recalled that he was sent to the "best" schools and was encouraged to achieve; he believed that the family had high expectations of him and that he received encouragement at each step. He followed his father's career and was very successful. The younger brother experienced his childhood as being chaotic and confusing and lacking in encouragement and nurturance. His school performance was below average, even though his tested intelligence was similar to his brother's. He had few friends, and by the time he finished high school he thought that he had been written off as a success in life. He married relatively young, but his low self-esteem and other personality problems led to marital difficulties and eventual divorce. Since then he has had difficulties forming meaningful relationships and in being able to develop career direction. The older sibling believed that he would "escape" HD, whereas the younger one was convinced that he would eventually become symptomatic.

FUNCTIONS OF PRESELECTION

The strategy of patient preselection serves several functions. First, it serves to contain and bind the family's anxiety about the threat of the genetic disorder. It provides the illusion of protection from the disease—it will happen to him, not to me. In essence, others buy the illusion of freedom at the expense of the preselected patient, who more and more functions as a "sacrificial lamb." In one family, the two at-risk siblings of a preselected person independently both averred that they *knew* that they would not get HD. On the other hand, the preselected patient was already convinced that he had HD symptoms even though frequent neurological examinations could not confirm it. Preselection helps to organize the family's experience of the disorder, and assigning the respective roles of the "healthy one" and the "sick one" enables most relatives to contain their fears and anxieties about becoming affected. Second, the strategy serves to resolve ambivalence toward the affected parent. The latter may be seen as a frightening, repugnant, and hated figure. At the same time, prior to the onset of symptoms, the affected parent may have been a source of love and attention and, in turn, was loved, admired, and idealized by the child. By projecting the negative feelings on the preselected person, the positive feelings for the affected person might be retained. Third, the preselected individual functions as a scapegoat for other nongenetic family problems. For example, focusing attention of the preselected individual and his or her behavior may deflect attention away from a marital dysfunction existing prior to the onset of symptoms in the affected parent or occurring with the advancing illness.

IMPACT ON THE PRESELECTED INDIVIDUAL

Being preselected generally has a profound impact on the individual's functioning. Frequently, the latter has major difficulties pulling his or her life together. In contrast to the encouragement and affirmation given to the other children, the preselected person's progress is often frustrated by the denial or withholding of adequate attention and resources. It is as if the family is saying, "Why waste our resources on someone who is going to become ill anyway?" In one instance, even though other adult relatives were available, a preselected adolescent was "assigned" the task of major caretaking of a severely affected widower father so that the older siblings could continue to pursue their educational and career paths. The latter went on to successful careers, whereas the preselected sibling had pervasive difficulties in these areas.

Some preselected individuals may have difficulty finishing their education or selecting and being successful at a chosen career. Generally they have low self-esteem and tend to suffer from periodic bouts of depression. There tends to be a negative mental set about the future that operates to undermine achievements and a sense of accomplishment. In some, there is a repetitive tendency to abort activities leading to success in school or work just at the point when such successes are at hand. Some live marginally in their social and economic activities and express a sense of not being worthy of the positive things life has to offer.

Some preselected relatives in families among whom HD occurs function virtually as if they already had symptoms of the disorder. They may show movements and mannerisms similar to those shown by their affected relatives, although it is a matter of mimicry. Their anticipation of becoming affected is often shown in the way they speak of themselves: "*When* I become affected" rather than "*If* I become affected." Also, their difficulties with life are frequently interpreted both by themselves and by their relatives as indicators or proofs of impending disease and thus have a reinforcing, self-perpetuating quality.

NONSELECTED RELATIVES

Since the chance of being affected with HD is random, individuals who are not preselected may have enormous difficulties adjusting to the reality that they may become or are becoming affected; it is not the way the script is supposed to be played out. Enormous resistance is shown to fend off the possibility that a non-preselected individual is showing symptoms. Visits to physicians may be put off and the entire family may collude to support the denial that may be necessary to keep the burgeoning symptoms of the disorder out of the individual's awareness.

FINAL REMARKS

Psychological changes seen in persons affected with HD are often ascribed to the disease process itself. However, such changes might also be due, either partially or entirely, to presymptomatic family dynamics. The attitudes and behaviors of caretakers and "significant others" may play an important role in shaping the suspiciousness, depression, and other symptoms often seen in persons with HD. The influence of the family system in promoting suicide among some persons affected with HD has been discussed (Kessler, 1987a, 1987b). The increasing sense of burden and helplessness among caretakers often leads to attitudes and behaviors to which affected individuals tend to respond with depression, despair, suicidal thoughts, and suicidal behaviors. Family dynamics are also shaped by social, cultural, and other influences. Professional pessimism about the lack of cure and adequate treatment of the disorder often affects the perceptions of patients and their relatives and may contribute to the avoidance of further professional contact, the discounting of professional advice, and the promotion of feelings of shame and stigma that pervade individual and family functioning. Societal attitudes toward the chronically ill and to their medical and long-term care reflect values and foster beliefs that influence individual attitudes and behavior. The paucity of adequate facilities for the long-term care of individuals affected with HD and the prospect of financial drain unsupported by societal willingness to provide for such catastrophic situations provides the backdrop for the shame, neglect, depression, and suicidal behaviors among affected individuals and their relatives. Thus, on many levels and in many ways systems factors and family dynamics influence the responses of persons affected with genetic disease and of their relatives. Greater understanding of these influences and dynamics is needed to increase the effectiveness of counseling or therapeutic work with families among whom HD and other genetic disorders occur. This is particularly important in preparing families for presymptomatic testing and providing later follow-up, since findings in one person can have important ramifications for others in the family.

REFERENCES

Kessler S (1987a) The dilemma of suicide and Huntington disease. Am J Med Genet 26:315–317.

Kessler S (1987b) Psychiatric implications of presymptomatic testing for Huntington's disease. Am J Orthopsychiatr 57:212–219.

Wexler NS (1979) Genetic "Russian roulette": the experience of being "at risk" for Huntington's disease. In: Kessler S (ed). Genetic Counseling: Psychological Dimensions. New York: Academic Press, pp 199–220.

6

Advanced Counseling Techniques[1]

INTRODUCTION

In my experience, genetic counselors often find that, with professional maturation, the procedures of personal counseling and psychotherapy tend to play a much larger role in their work than they did when they first entered the field. This process seems to parallel a common phenomenon in other fields of personal counseling, namely that, regardless of their initial theoretical position or the school of thought to which they adhere, experienced counselors and psychotherapists tend to come to resemble one another in their actual work (Karasu, 1992). These professionals tend to find that certain procedures or techniques seem to work in helping clients solve their problems and live more effective lives. In this paper I would like to address four such techniques that genetic counselors might find useful in their counseling efforts: interview procedures, clarifying procedures, reframing, and role playing.

INTERVIEW PROCEDURES

Many experienced counselors and psychotherapists tend to use relatively simple interview techniques, which show a commonality in that the professional comes across as *less* knowledgeable, *less* certain, and *less* authoritative than he or she is in reality. Conclusions and interpretations are presented in provisional ways, hedged, so that the

[1]This essay first appeared as Kessler S (1997) Psychological aspects of genetic counseling. X. Advanced counseling techniques. *Journal of Genetic Counseling* 6:379–392. Reprinted with kind permission of the publisher, Kluwer Academic/Human Sciences Press.

door to other as yet unrevealed possibilities is kept open. For example, they might ask questions or make statements in the following way:

- *I'm not sure* I know what you mean when you say you don't believe in abortion?
- *Correct me if I'm wrong* but you *seem* to want the amnio procedure. I'm not sure how you [to spouse] feel about it?
- *I may be wrong* but what I *think* you're saying is that you do not want to continue this pregnancy.
- *I wonder* how you understand that?

In each case, the professional uses a formulation in which he or she appears tentative about what conclusions to draw from the information given by the client. I wish to underscore the word *appears*, since often the professional may have a good idea of what the client is saying, yet chooses to "play dumb" for several reasons. First, this strategy encourages the emergence of new information. The professional proceeds on the premise that clients often do not give us a full picture of a situation and that the information they do provide often tends to be partial and minimizes or distorts their perceived failings and faults. Anyone who has worked with couples knows that the same set of events might be portrayed differently and assigned differing meanings by each partner (Kessler, 1996a). Thus, the professional attempts to avoid or minimize drawing premature conclusions and coming to total closure on any given issue. Lipp (1977), Cassell (1985), and others admonish us to remember that no matter how open a person is, they always have information about themselves that the professional does not have.

Second, this strategy gives the client the message that the professional is interested in understanding them. This facilitates the building of rapport and trust and contributes to a sense of mutuality between the professional and client.

Third, the strategy helps clients clarify their thinking in an effort to explain themselves to the professional. This has an additional advantage in that it encourages the client to talk more. In turn, this has a cascade effect in which by increasing the client's participation in the session, it promotes the feeling that they have greater control over what is going on, which tends to reinforce or increase their sense of autonomy and self-directedness.

Fourth, the strategy humanizes the professional by making him or her appear more fallible and less authoritative than he or she may actually be. This is especially important in genetic counseling, where the goal generally is to help the client make autonomous decisions. The tendency for professionals to emphasize their authority—either by advice-giving, playing the educator role, or not identifying with the client—often impedes their decision making and defeats the achievement of nondirective goals (Kessler, 1996b).

Some counselors and therapists almost make a point of portraying themselves as less than perfect. The family therapist Salvador Minuchen once described how he began work with a family in which the identified patient was a teenage girl with anorexia. He entered the room, sat down, and promptly knocked over the contents of a full ashtray that was on a side table. Considerable apologies and bumbling followed.

He might not have purposely planned that action but, nonetheless, it made the point that we are all human and thus prone to make mistakes, an issue that became the focus of the ensuing therapy.

In establishing rapport, the professional has an opportunity to assess how the client uses language to communicate. Some clients describe their experiences in terms of manipulations or motoric imagery (e.g., I can't *get a handle* on the problem) whereas others may use sensory images (e.g., I *see* what you mean; I *hear* what you're saying). Experienced counselors adjust their language to "match" that of the client and by doing so create images with words that the client can access readily, thus facilitating communication.

One of the effective ways of establishing rapport with another person is to show appropriate interest in them. "Where did you get those beautiful earrings?" "Oh, what a pretty dress!" "That haircut is very becoming." "Oh, you like murder mysteries too! Who are your favorite authors?" These are some of the myriad ways of expressing interest in someone else, effective especially when combined with a compliment to the person.

In a profession that attempts to promote the client's ability to make their own decisions, a necessary counseling strategy would be to highlight evidence of their competence and to provide positive reinforcement to any tendency toward self-directedness and autonomy. Early on in a counseling session, experienced professionals identify key areas of client functioning, which they use throughout the session to strengthen the latter's sense of competence. This might involve parenting, work, interpersonal, or other issues and requires the professional to say rewarding things to the client.

Some genetic counselors, especially in the early stages of their careers, tend to be niggardly in praising and commending their clients out of the mistaken belief to do so would diminish their professionalism. One possible reason for this is that in their training they were exposed to psychodynamic ideas that actively discourage the gratification of such wishes. The truth is, clients almost always crave the approval, high regard, and respect of professionals. Furthermore, in giving praise for overcoming obstacles, standing up to authority (even if it is the counselor or his or her colleagues), showing good judgment, being competent, etc., the counselor reinforces such behaviors. Some simple examples follow:

- "Oh, that was clever of you!"
- "You've had to deal with a lot of very difficult situations and you've done so really well."
- "I admire you for how well you handled that doctor."
- "That's a great question!"
- "It's so wonderful to watch you with your baby; there's so much caring and love."
- "You really know how to do it!"

A common mistake made by beginning counselors is to try to explain or make excuses for the actions of other professionals. (e.g., "Oh, I'm sure he didn't mean to hurt your feelings" or "She was probably having an off day.") Thus, rather than trying to "cover" for, let us say, your medical geneticist employer, it might be more productive to say something to the effect: "Well, you sure know what you need or want when you talk to a doctor" or some other statement that keeps you from mediating between the client and the professional and, simultaneously, rewards the client for assertiveness and autonomy. Generally when clients tell you something negative about some other professional, they are testing you to see how you will react.

When the professional is on the receiving end of criticism, it becomes more difficult to avoid being defensive and yet, with practice, it is not only possible, it is crucial for the client's sake. Once, following a rather stormy session with a client, she returned the following week and berated me in no uncertain terms for being insensitive and "a complete jerk." Rather than become defensive or attempt to explain myself and clarify misunderstandings—strategies that might have invalidated and dismissed the client's feelings and end up making her feel blamed for what occurred—I took the opportunity to swallow my pride and agreed with her. I told her that I was in the wrong and that I felt sorry. I went on to say, "What I did was inexcusable and was exactly what your father might have said and done in similar circumstances," etc. Whatever other thoughts and feelings I had at that moment were deliberately suppressed so that I could help the client see the re-enactment aspects of a situation for which the client was invariably blamed in the past. It also validated her expression of strong feelings and gave the message that I could withstand them and survive. If the goal is to promote the client's self-esteem and autonomy, genetic counselors need to be psychologically capable of receiving criticism when the former "dish it out."

Experienced professionals rarely give advice; they do so when it is clear that the advice would promote the autonomy of the client and only after understanding the client in a full, deep way (which might be possible in psychotherapy but seldom in genetic counseling). Also, when they do give advice, it is generally in the form of suggestions that they make clear can be rejected fully or in part by the client (Kessler, 1996b).

Clarifying Procedures

Genetic counselors with limited experience tend to hear requests for direct advice literally and, frequently, because their counseling skills have not matured (or possibly out of other ego needs), respond by actually giving it. Generally forgotten in the process is that advice-giving is often a vote of no confidence in the client's own ability to sort things out for themselves and arrive at their own conclusions. It needs to be remembered that most of the people seen for genetic counseling are experienced decision-makers; they have already made multiple decisions in the course of their lives without our help.

Experienced professionals seldom interpret requests for advice literally and tend to hear them rather as requests for a piece of information the client seems to lack that would help them make their own decision. Commonly, this information concerns a way to think about a problem rather than a solution.

Experienced professionals tend to assist clients in thinking through problems by providing a framework by which the client might see the nature of the problem more clearly. Essentially, they take the client's own thinking and, so-to-speak, clean it up so that its core becomes apparent. For example, in response to a confused advanced maternal age client who asks, "What would you advise your sister to do in this situation?" the following might be said: "I suppose if my sister had turned to me for advice I would ask her the same questions I would ask you. How would she feel if she didn't have the amniocentesis and then had a child with a genetic problem? Would she be able to live with it and with herself, or would she berate herself for the rest of her life? Also, I would ask her what she might do if she had the amnio and we found that the fetus had a genetic problem? What would she do then? How do you feel about these issues?"

The professional in this situation has taken the client's dilemma and, presumably, her verbal and nonverbal communications and voiced them without giving advice about the ultimate decision she should make. *This procedure is the core of nondirective counseling.* It also should be noted that the structure of the reply to the client's question implies that the professional would deal with her as if she were his or her own sister, thus reducing the emotional distance between them and de-emphasizing the issue of authority (while simultaneously maintaining it).

Another example relevant to genetic counseling would be a response to such direct questions for advice as, "What would you do in my place?" A counselor might say the following: "I really don't know what I'd do in your place, but I can tell you how I might think about it. There's part of me that would be saying I want another child and I want it to be healthy and another part that's afraid that if I did have a child it would be one with a problem and that's not what I want. So I guess I would have to ask myself am I ready and willing to take the risk to have a child knowing that there are no guarantees in life. What are your thoughts about that?"

Here again, the professional focuses on the *thinking* process clients might use to come to their own decision. Rather than give advice, he or she provides a framework by means of which the clients might reach their own decision. When clients have obvious difficulties in clarifying their own thinking—a problem often seen among persons experiencing stress and anxiety—providing a way of thinking a problem through is often welcomed and perceived as helpful.

It is important to remember that this clarifying procedure needs to be adapted to the general cognitive style of the client. Counseling differs from other interactions in that it is the professional's obligation to adjust his or her style to that of the client, not vice versa. Rather than employ a one-style-fits-all approach, the counselor may need to determine what style of thinking might best fit a particular client's needs and use the framework that accommodates the client's way of thinking. The approach suggested here is not incompatible with the views of Kenen and Smith (1995), Brunger and Lippman (1995), and others.

Experienced professionals pay special attention to the language a client uses to describe a given situation or problem. A problem described as a "disaster" is generally given a differing inner representation and emotional valence than one described as a "bruise." When these representations or valences interfere with problem solving and other adaptive activities, professionals often attempt to modify the client's perceptions by substituting language that possibly evokes more productive meanings and images. Related to this technique is one in which counselors and psychotherapists reduce complex larger problems—ones clients often describe as overwhelming—into smaller, more manageable steps.

For example, take the following brief scenario with a couple discussing the possibility of having an amniocentesis:

1. Mother: I want it.
2. Father: I don't believe in abortion. Well, what are we going to do?

An experienced genetic counselor might break down the disagreement between the couple into two or more separate steps as follows: At (2), for example, the counselor might say: "I'm not sure what you mean when you say you don't *believe* in abortion," and thus obtain clarification of what the father has in mind, the limits of his objection, etc. In other words, the flexibility or "give" in the system would be explored; perhaps the couple is not that far apart in their respective opinions. On the other hand, the counselor might discover that the father feels so strongly about abortion he might abandon his mate over it. Imagine if the professional discovers this after he or she has already given advice!

An alternative approach the genetic counselor might use in the previous situation would be to separate the issue of having an amniocentesis from that of having an abortion by saying at (2): "You know, having an amniocentesis does not obligate or commit you to have an abortion." The counselor might then be able to help the couple deal with their thinking about knowing the health status of the fetus in advance and ascertain what differences of opinion exist, if any. He or she might then explore what meaning the partners give to not knowing the status of the fetus in advance.

REFRAMING

Another strategy experienced counselors and psychotherapists often use is that of reframing, which refers to the reformulation of an issue in a way different than the one originally presented. The reformulation serves to open or expand inherent possibilities not immediately apparent to the client.

In general, individuals and couples come to a professional with a relatively constricted way of assessing and assigning meaning to the problem that motivated them to seek counseling. These formulations are frequently part of the reason why they have not been able to find a satisfactory solution on their own. In reframing, the professional helps the clients see their problems from a different perspective, one which possibly offers them an opportunity to also see novel solutions.

One of the classic reframing strategies frequently used in family therapy is the redefinition of a child's acting-out behavior, such as fire-setting or a suicidal gesture, as a cry for (professional) help. The act, although unpleasant and disturbing for everyone involved, often brings the child and the family to professional attention and thus opens the potentiality of receiving assistance and guidance. Thus, an act with a negative connotation, which ordinarily might evoke hostility, punishment, and longer-term resentment, is transformed into an action with the potential for enormous long-term positivity.

In genetic counseling, there are multiple opportunities to use reframing techniques. For example, in taking pedigree information clients often make gratuitous comments about certain relatives and the quality of various relationships. After describing his parents and siblings, one client said, "I'm the dummy of the family." And so I asked him, "Why do you say that?" He replied, "Well all through my childhood, every time I said something or did anything, my father rolled his eyes and said, 'That was a dumb thing to do.' " Based on the information he had already provided, I asked him, "Could it be that your father was in competition with you and that might have been his way of keeping you in a one-down position?" The client replied, "I never thought of it that way, but it feels right."

A timely reframing intervention may help change a perception charged with a negative valence to one that might either be neutral or positive and may have a long-term impact on counselees. In the course of describing her family constellation, one client began to complain about her mother's persistent controlling behavior. I asked her in what way did her mother control her, and she replied that ever since she told her mother she was going to take the predictive test for Huntington disease (HD), the latter telephoned her each day. I then asked her whether or not her mother was an anxious lady and she said, "She must hold the world's record!" I then offered that perhaps her mother was calling her as a way of reassuring herself that the client was still all right rather than as a way of controlling her. In other words, she was behaving that way as a means of controlling herself (and her own emotions) rather than the client. The latter took it in and was silent for a few moments and slowly, tears began to form in the corners of her eyes. Finally, she said, "I guess she does really care about me."

Situations involving loss occasionally offer opportunities for reframing. For example, in trying to reach a decision about an abortion, some clients are captured by the thought and feelings associated with the forthcoming loss. They might focus on the lost opportunity to provide a sibling for a child, the loss of the pleasure of carrying or completing a pregnancy, etc. Reframing takes advantage of the fact that most losses have another side; they make room for other things, other relationships, learning important life lessons, etc.

Reframing is especially useful when interpersonal conflict is involved. Once in the course of a HD support group meeting, the issue of reproduction was brought up by a person at-risk for the disorder. After some heated discussion, two schools of thought emerged, one favoring reproduction in spite of the genetic risk and the other opposing it, arguing that it was an irresponsible action. Since neutrality on the leader's part was desirable, it was prudent to reframe the discussion in a way that left each side feeling understood and valued. Thus, it was pointed out that not long ago at the height of the Cold War, many young couples felt it was foolhardy and perhaps irresponsible to have children because of the nuclear threat hanging over the human species. Many of their friends were having children and it was likely that there were family and cultural pressures to have a family. Thus, to decide not to have children required courage to stand up for what one believed. On the other hand, some couples felt that they needed to have faith in tomorrow and in the continuation of the species. In other words, they needed to believe that the world would become a better place, if not in their lifetime, then in their children's. One needed courage to believe that at a time when the future looked so bleak. It took courage in both situations. In short, the issue of reproduction was reformulated in terms of human courage and the necessity of acting courageously regardless of one's choice. Each side of the argument felt supported and it broadened the scope of the issue from one facing individuals at-risk for a genetic disorder to one that was part of the general human condition.[2]

The use of reframing to deal with some issues of guilt has been discussed by Kessler et al. (1984). For example, expressions of personal responsibility for a child's genetic problems, in appropriate cases, might be dealt with by taking advantage of the fact that the word *responsibility* has more than one meaning: responsibility, hence guilt for a problem as opposed to responsibility, hence competency and trustworthiness. In some instances, cognitive information may help reframe perceptions and thus reduce guilt (Chapple et al., 1995).

Reframing can be used in conjunction with other counseling procedures. For instance, a few months ago, I saw a woman who said to me she needed help dealing with her older sister. The woman, a successful professional, gave birth to a child with multiple cardiac defects and a unilateral cleft lip and palate. The child needed enormous caretaking. During the period in which I saw her, the child had undergone three or four major life-threatening surgeries. Her sister was helpful during this period and often baby-sat for her so that she and her husband could occasionally get out of the house. Now the sister was asking her to reciprocate and wanted my client to baby-sit for her for an evening. My client did not want to do so and focused on the possibility that her sister's child might have head lice and she didn't want her child to become infected. She didn't know whether to reciprocate or to turn her sister down and suffer the possible consequences of causing a rift between the two of them. I listened to her and said something along the following lines:

> "You know Mary, you are a very giving person. And when you give you do so all the way. Now under normal circumstances you have plenty of energy to put out to others, and when you do, you have plenty of reserves to replenish the energy you expend. But what you've gone through over the past 9 months has depleted all your reserves. The tanks are on empty, so that any demand, even a small one, anyone makes feels enormous and you end up feeling that you will be totally drained if you give even a little of your energy. Under normal circumstances I'm sure you'd be able to find a way to accommodate your sister, but after all you've gone through, you're exhausted. You haven't been living under normal circumstances for so long now, you feel you have barely enough energy for yourself no less for someone else."

As soon as I said these things I saw the pain on my client's face dissipate and her body relax because she knew I understood what she was going through. Notice, I did

---

[2]Shifting attention from one's personal problems or perspective to one with broader or universal meaning is a way of making therapeutic interventions, particularly in support groups. Many such groups often reinforce a tendency to invest participants' narcissistic energies into one's particular disorder or dysfunction and thus do not help the person heal and find transcending meaning in their life problems.

not attempt to solve the client's dilemma; it would have been presumptuous of me to have attempted to do so especially since I had no idea of what I could suggest. Thus, I tried to reframe the situation in a way that let her know that her feelings were reasonable and that, in general, almost any problem she would face would present difficulties since she was coming from a place of exhaustion. This also helped her clarify her thinking so that she could go on to decide whatever it was she had to do.

ROLE-PLAYING

Role-playing is a procedure in which participants pretend they are coping with a specific person or situation and play-act or rehearse different approaches and solutions. It allows the client to experience what it might feel like to make a specific decision, be in a specific situation, or be someone else, and is thus a powerful educational and counseling technique. For example, a parent may be unsure how to inform their child about the presence of a genetic disorder in the family. The counselor and client might role-play that situation, the former, let us say, taking the part of the child who needs to be informed. In one such instance, a man who had just ascertained his gene status through predictive testing for HD wanted to inform his adolescent son about his at-risk status and was uncertain how to go about doing it. After some discussion I asked him to pretend that I was his son and imagine we are taking a walk in a park on a Sunday morning. I asked him to take a deep breath and plunge in and tell me what was on his mind. After an initial fumble, he finally broke the news to me, however, it was done crudely and in a somewhat heavy-handed way. This was pointed out to him and so he tried a second time and was more successful in conveying his thoughts. However, the right tone had not been achieved. Thus, I suggested that we reverse roles; I would be him and he would be his son. In this configuration I was able to suggest how he might convey the information more sensitively and tactfully. It only required the provision of a key word or phrase that he had overlooked.

Another instance where role-playing was used was with a divorced mother of a young adolescent child who wanted to tell him about the fact that his father was affected with HD. In a roleplay she blurted out, "Your father has this terrible disease called Huntington's, and he's going to die and you are going to get it too" and she broke into sobs. Obviously such an approach was doomed to maximize the trauma to the child and would have been counterproductive. Role-playing helped her find a more appropriate formula and a more effective approach. Hearing herself say the words several times in practice made the task less fearful and less overwhelming and helped her contain her emotions so as to leave room for the child to ask questions or express his own feelings.

Role-playing may be helpful for couples in the throes of decision making. It may help mates who disagree with one another see the other person's point of view with greater empathy. For example, I worked briefly with a couple who needed to make a decision whether or not to abort a fetus found to have a trisomy. The couple already had two healthy children and this was probably their last chance to have another baby. The husband was adamant about having the abortion, but the wife resisted. After some lengthy discussion, they both seemed entrenched in their respective viewpoints and so I asked them whether or not they wished to role-play the dilemma. They both agreed eagerly. It was only when the husband placed himself—so to speak—in his wife's shoes, that he realized how important this pregnancy had been for her; she had waited so long for this ultimate pregnancy and now that it had happened, she felt that nothing would come of it if she lost it through an abortion. It was an emotional moment for both of them after which she confessed that she knew all along that she would abort this fetus. However, she had felt so hurt that no one, neither the professionals she dealt with nor her husband, had given her even a token word of congratulation or well-wishes on the pregnancy; she simply could not end it.

DISCUSSION

Because the profession holds itself out to the public as genetic counseling, a not unreasonable expectation is that professionals will be capable of applying quality counseling skills. Given the paucity of information about the process of genetic counseling, the extent to which this accords with reality is not known. A superficial reading of the pertinent literature suggests that there might be considerable room for improvement.

Elsewhere (Kessler, 1997), the differences between the professional attitudes, underlying philosophies, and methods of educational and counseling activities were discussed. Genetic counselors often try to combine aspects of both approaches only to find that their respective goals often conflict with one another and tend to cancel each other out. It would be an extremely rare individual who could realistically develop a practice-based competency in all the areas outlined in recently adopted standards (Fine et al., 1996) of the genetic counseling profession. Moreover, considerable skill and flexibility is required to accomplish one goal no less than two very different ones. The net result, in my opinion, has been an overemphasis on teaching or communication at the expense of developing and refining counseling skills. Thus, as genetic counselors mature professionally, they often find themselves handicapped by a lack of training and experience in the attitudes and skills of personal counselors, skills, which once acquired, often transform their work and give it a richer personal meaning. Difficulties in achieving and maintaining a nondirective stance may result from inadequacies in such attitudes and skills (Kessler, 1996b).

In the training of genetic counselors, there has been an overriding emphasis on so-called Rogerian and client-centered techniques. It seems to be assumed that such procedures, by themselves, are adequate for genetic counseling purposes. This, in my opinion, is a gross misunderstanding of the applicability of procedures designed primarily for long-term psychotherapy to the short-term context of genetic counseling. The generally short duration of professional–client contact, economic constraints, the predominate focus on genetic problems, as well as a need to minimize transferential reactions all argue against an over-reliance on reflective Rogerian techniques or procedures that limit the problem-solving functions of the counselor. Helping clients, in the time available, make sense of information, make decisions, and deal with psychological reactions requires a more active counseling stance than that needed in long-term psychotherapy.

Unfortunately, genetic counseling students largely have been taught to be active teachers, but passive counselors. For example, the development of listening skills is overly stressed in their training, whereas the acquisition of active response skills tends to be neglected. This, in combination with many other factors, tends to promote a sense of inadequacy in applying counseling skills. Being a "good listener" by itself does not a counselor make. Effective counselors have learned what to listen to and what to listen for and what meaning it has. In addition, they do more than listen, they act.

Similarly, the continued emphasis on "being supportive" neglects to teach students what is necessary to support and what is not, what one actively reinforces and what one ignores or actively extinguishes. Effective counselors do not support behaviors in an unqualified way. They are highly selective, supporting clients by reinforcing behaviors that promote the latter's interests and autonomy and actively discouraging those that do not. In my opinion, the repeated emphasis on being a "good listener" and of providing "support"—the most superficial aspects of counseling—as hallmarks of a genetic counselor are ways of inculcating passivity, ensuring ineffectiveness, and impeding the acquisition and development of quality counseling skills.

The need for less passivity among genetic counselors is imperative and the procedures discussed here all require genetic counselors to be active in their counseling role. Passivity may reduce the perceived emotional risks for individual counselors but it also impedes the maturation and refinement of their counseling skills.

Genetic counselors are helping professionals and, in real terms, the provision of help requires active, appropriate involvement with clients. Involvement, in turn, requires the reduction of the "counseling distance" between professionals and clients and an elimination of psychological barriers so that the counselor's humanity, with all its strengths and fallibilities, becomes clearly visible.

ACKNOWLEDGMENT

I dedicate this article to a friend and a major leader in the training of genetic counselors, Ms. Joan Marks.

REFERENCES

Brunger F, Lippman A (1995) Resistance and adherence to the norms of genetic counseling. J Genet Counsel 4:151–167.

Cassell EJ (1985) Talking with Patients. Vol. 1: The Theory of Doctor–Patient Communication. Cambridge, MA: MIT Press

Chapple A, May C, Campion P (1995) Parental guilt: the part played by the clinical geneticist. J Genet Counsel 4:179–191.

Fine BA, Baker DL, Fiddler M (1996) Practice-based competencies for accreditation of and training in graduate programs in genetic counseling. J Genet Counsel 5:113–121.

Karasu TB (1992) Wisdom in the Practice of Psychotherapy. New York: Basic Books.

Kenen RH, Smith ACM (1995) Genetic counseling for the next 25 years: models for the future. J Genet Counsel 4:115–124.

Kessler S (1996a) Health issues in couples therapy. In: Kessler H (ed). Couples Therapy. San Francisco: Jossey-Bass, pp 137–163.

Kessler S (1996b) Nondirectiveness revisited. Talk given at National Society of Genetic Counselors 15th Annual Educational Conference, San Francisco, October, 27, 1996.

Kessler S (1997) Psychological aspects of genetic counseling. IX. Teaching and counseling. J Genet Counsel 6:287–295.

Kessler S, Kessler H, Ward P (1984) Psychological aspects of genetic counseling. III. Management of guilt and shame. Am J Med Genet 171:673–697.

Lipp MR (1977) Respectful Treatment: The Human Side of Medical Care. Hagerstown, MD: Harper & Row.

7

More on Counseling Skills[1]

On rare occasions the lid lifts and we are granted a fleeting glimpse into the black box of genetic counseling. What we view generally are human beings interacting and striving to understand one another. We try to overhear a few of the words they exchange and realize that they do not always seem to be speaking a common language. Their assumptions about things seem vastly different and there are other impediments to communication and mutual understanding.

The professionals in these colloquies often seem resolved to talk about certain specific matters, numbers, and statistics, for example, regardless of whatever else might be happening in the counseling interaction. Some seem to have an overriding agenda of educating the clients about the complex world of human genetics. On their part, the latter do not always seem to be certain about what they want from the professionals; their motives, wishes, thoughts, and feelings seem complex and unclear, perhaps even to themselves. Communication in the session can be labored, opaque, indirect, at times incomprehensible. Clients have difficulty making themselves understood; professionals have difficulty understanding them. The result is a misdirection of efforts.

Research on genetic counseling rarely looks at this reality. Generally, most studies focus on outcome measures such as an increase in knowledge, changes in reproductive intentions, or client satisfaction. Overall, these studies suggest that there is considerable room for improvement, which is a kindly way of stating that the "process of communication" is less than a smashing success. The few studies concerning the process of genetic counseling also reveal considerable inadequacies in the counseling

[1]This essay first appeared as Kessler S (1998) Psychological aspects of genetic counseling. XII. More on counseling skills. *Journal of Genetic Counseling* 7:263–278. Reprinted with kind permission of the publisher, Kluwer Academic/Human Sciences Press.

skills of genetic counselors (Kelly, 1977; Kessler, 1979, 1981; Kessler and Jacopini, 1982; Michie et al., 1997). Problems in such skills contribute to difficulties in achieving or sustaining nondirective goals (Kessler, 1997a, 1997b). Also, analyses of transcripts of genetic counseling (Kessler, 1997c) reveal major shortcomings in building rapport with clients, understanding what the latter are saying, and providing empathy. A case can be made that the level of basic counseling skills among practitioners of genetic counseling need considerable improvement.

In the present paper further examples will be given of situations in which genetic counselors seem to run into difficulties in applying their counseling skills. Suggestions will be made to help counselors understand the nature of these problems and how they might deal with such situations more effectively. In the examples below I will summarize the interactions between clients and professionals, analyze the situation from the psychological perspective and provide some comments on the professionals' interventions. Each line of the transcript will be numbered so that the reader can refer back to the points in the analysis and commentary. The goals here are to stimulate further discussion, help professionals improve their skills and provide teachers of genetic counselors a way of thinking about the training of their students.

EXAMPLE 1

This example[2] is a hypothetical scenario that appeared as an illustration of dialogical counseling (White, 1997). It concerns a woman who has apparently just received her amniocentesis results in which a fetus with Down syndrome was identified. The woman's husband is not present at the session and we are not told whether or not he has been informed about the prenatal test results. The professional (P) is about "to explore the client's (C) feelings about the diagnosis."

1. P: In order to help you make your decision whether or not to
2. continue your pregnancy, there are a number of things I'd
3. like to make sure we discuss. If there are any issues you
4. would rather not talk about please say so, but my goal is to
5. be sure you have a good grasp of what Down syndrome may mean
6. for you as a parent, and that we have explored the range of
7. factors that commonly contribute to those kinds of
8. decisions. Is that all right with you?
9. C: Sure.
10. P: Have you thought about the kinds of expectations you have
11. for your children?
12. C: I always imagined I'd have several children, and hoped
13. for nothing more than that they would be happy, have lots of

[2]Used by permission of Human Sciences Press.

EXAMPLE 1   **87**

14. of friends and be successful in whatever they decided to do.
15. P: How do you think you might feel if you had a child who
16. might not finish high school?
17. C: I'd be sad, I guess for him that is, but so long as he is
18. happy I think I would feel ok. Every person is different,
19. some are smarter than others, not everyone can be a college
20. graduate. Sure, I know some people think children that are
21. retarded shouldn't be born; they would abort this baby.
22. But, for me, this is my child, a person—abortion would be
23. like killing my own child.
24. P: We have talked about the special needs of children with
25. Down syndrome. Do you feel you are prepared for those
26. needs?
27. C: Well, I guess you're never really prepared even for a normal
28. child. But I think I and my husband will be good parents.
29. Most of all, we want a chance to share our love with another
30. person, to watch our child grow, to have the experience of
31. being parents. But, I am nervous . . . This is a hard
32. decision—what would you do?
33. [*After disclaiming that she shares the same values as C, P*
34. *gives advice to terminate the pregnancy.*]
35. [*C responds by saying things she believes will please P.*]

Summary

P concentrates on the decision to continue or terminate the pregnancy (1–8). She tells C she has an agenda of issues that she feels they need to discuss. She focuses attention on C's expectations for her children (10–11); these may be hypothetical ones since we do not know whether or not C has children in "reality." C responds in a somewhat Pollyanna-ish, perhaps guarded way (12–14). P pursues the line of possible disappointment C might experience if her child is retarded (15–16). C picks up on P's metamessage and states her values regarding abortion (20–23). P asks whether C feels prepared to deal with a child with problems (25–26) and C says that no one can really be prepared for such things (27–28) and that she has apprehensions about it (31–32). She asks P for her opinion (32) and P gives it (33).

Analysis

From the onset P has an agenda of issues (2, 6) she wants to concentrate on. The central issue is abortion (1–2, 7–8); she is either going to sell it or not. On the surface it seems that she gives C a choice in the matter of the agenda (3–4), but the manner in which it is presented leaves C little choice but to assent (9). Rather than inquire about C's thinking at this point, P asks a very general question about C's expectations for children (10–11). The question is vague and C does not seem to know where P is coming from. Thus she responds to it in a general, vague way (12–14). She talks about happiness, a good social life, and success, (socially correct) terms that convey little substance and reveal nothing about underlying feelings; she seems guarded since P has not yet shown her hand. P then picks up on the issue of success and inquires how C might feel if her child failed to succeed intellectually (15–16). C replies in a guarded way (17–20) but then catches on to the possibility that P is pushing her to abort the pregnancy (20–21). She expresses her feelings about P's position in a rather strong way (22–23). P ignores her affect and without any expression of empathy moves back to her agenda emphasizing the special needs of children with Down syndrome (24–26). Her question implies that C is not prepared to deal with those needs. C backs down (27) and her ambivalence begins to emerge (31–32); she may feel that she and P are in conflict. C can argue with P if she wishes, but she may need her counsel (and approval) too much to do that. The safest strategy for C to follow is to appear compliant (27–31) and let P play out her agenda. She does this by asking P to get to the bottom line, "What would you do?" and then by saying things she believes might placate P (35). P comes down on the side of the ambivalence favoring abortion (33).

Comments

P seems less interested in C's feelings or thinking than in pursuing her own agenda. Her choice of an opening question (10–11) is the kind many attorneys—obtaining sworn testimony—refer to as "leading the person down the garden path." All of the questions appear benign but they steadily lead the person into a cul-de-sac in which positions stated earlier or convictions previously held are stealthily undermined. In my opinion this is a strategy of entrapment and has aspects of deception and thus should be considered as directive counseling (Kessler, 1997b). The person is given to believe that their responses to questions are in their own interest. It turns out that they are being ensnared in a situation in which the professional might impose her thinking. This is an accepted strategy in the legal system that operates on an adversarial basis, but as a counseling strategy it leaves a lot to be desired.

P's counseling skills in this illustration are both rudimentary and skillful. The questions she asks seem to have no foundation on which to build or to reveal the client's thinking to herself. They tend to convey a metamessage of, "You don't know what you're doing or what you're getting into." Thus they are intended to undermine C's autonomy and self-confidence and they appear to do so. Everything seems to lead to the same focal point, and that is to induce the question that allows P to give her advice.

The unlikely assumption of the excerpt is that the client is a blank slate and has neither given any thought to the issues on P's mind nor has she formulated a plan beforehand to deal with adverse results. If this is true, P might have done better to ascertain this more clearly. It would appear that there had been no preprocedural counseling.

EXAMPLE 2   **89**

The excerpt also proceeds on the premise that the advice P gives will be helpful, but given that we do not know how C's mate and broader social support system feel about all the issues, this is a risky counseling strategy. Moreover, when we read what P finally says to C, "I would choose to terminate this pregnancy" (White, 1997) it seems apparent that P has been less interested in exploring C's values than in stating and imposing her own. P admits that she and C do not share pertinent values (33). Thus, in what way would knowing what P might do help the latter? If anything, it may make decision making for C and her mate more difficult. If they do share values, why put C through the (in my way of thinking, disrespectful) exercise of pushing her into a corner?

How would a counselor with some skill deal with the situation at 32–35? The issue to recognize is that C has moved from a position of clarity and resolve (20–23) to one of ambivalence. An experienced counselor might recognize that his or her own coolness or lack of empathy (24–26) to what C had said (20–23) may have undermined the latter's autonomous position. This awareness might lead to more careful interventions. Also, the counselor would recognize that to support one side of C's ambivalent feelings before dealing with the nature of the ambivalence itself will probably not be helpful to C. I would have asked C at 31, 32, "What makes the decision so hard for you?" so that there would be greater clarity—both for P and C—as to what the conflict might be.

Sharing personal values may look good in the abstract, but it neither deals with the client's conflicts nor makes psychological sense. If the conflict has been generated by the professional, as in the example above, leaving the field of conflict would allow the client to return to her original position or to continue to oscillate between the two poles of her ambivalence. What then has P gained by sharing her values except perhaps some ego-gratification (Kessler, 1997a)? The client may have gained very little if anything.

EXAMPLE 2

In this excerpt (Kelly, 1977)[3], a couple is being interviewed by a female genetic counselor (C) a year after the husband (M) was diagnosed with Alport syndrome. At the time of diagnosis the couple apparently decided to have an amniocentesis in a future pregnancy. Attending the current meeting is M's wife (W) who is pregnant; apparently this is a routine follow-up visit.

1. M: Now you want to get our rationale? We both feel like
2. guilty children because we spent so much time talking with
3. you about amniocentesis. In the last couple of months,
4. prior to her becoming pregnant. . . .
5. W: Prior to trying, we made the decision. . . .
6. M: Our feeling, in a nutshell, is that we don't feel that

[3]Used by permission of Springer-Verlag New York, Inc.

7. the disease . . . [symptoms] are so severe looking at them 20–25
8. years in the future, that we really wish to interfere with
9. the natural course of this childbirth.
10. C: I'm interested in the term you used, that you feel like
11. guilty children.
12. M: Well, I say that because when we saw you a few months
13. ago, I thought we had pretty much committed ourselves to
14. amniocentesis, and just interpersonally we had an
15. understanding of what we were doing. And I think a lot has
16. happened in the meantime that you're not aware of.
17. C: I see. So in other words, if we discuss something a year
18. ago almost, and that's how you feel a year ago, somehow
19. you're supposed to stick by that over the next year!?
20. W: [*Continues to justify their decision and ends by saying:*]
21. [I]t's like somebody's given you advice and you've accepted
22. it initially and then you say, . . . "Thank you . . . but no
23. thanks."

Summary

M's initial statement (1) implies that he owes an explanation to C and needs to justify his decision. He suggests (2) that he and W have reneged on what they took as an agreement previously made with C. W enters to concur with M (5) who continues to justify their decision; she implies that their decision was made not long after their initial meeting with C. C focuses on M's term guilty children (11). M then elaborates on their thinking and continues to justify their decision (12–16). C attempts to say something to the effect that it is all right for them to change their minds (17–19). However, it does not seem to make much impact since W provides further justification for their decision (20–23). She implies that C had advised them to use amniocentesis and on reflection they decided to reject her advice.

Analysis

The excerpt begins as if C had asked the clients a question about their decision; it is doubtful that she did. This gives greater force to M's justifications; it is self-initiated (1) and immediately becomes clear that the central psychological issue here is largely that of transference. This issue dominates the discussion to the very end of the excerpt. M's use of the terms you (1 and again at 3), interpersonally (14), and guilty children (2) all point to the difficulties the clients seem to have with C. Insufficient information is available as to how C herself evaluated this situation in her own mind although the context in which the excerpt is presented suggests that she focused on the issue of decision making rather than on the transferential one.

EXAMPLE 2   **91**

The term guilty children (2) captures C's attention, as I imagine it would for the majority of genetic counselors. Her statement (10) reflects her interest and presumably is intended to draw the clients out, so that they might elaborate either on why they feel guilty or why they feel like children. The phrasing of the statement however implies a clinical detachment—a curiosity—rather than a desire for a closer engagement with the clients. The phrasing also seems to imply that she is not aware that she is the target of the client's projections and feelings.

In her second statement (17–19), the professional is trying to say to the clients that it's O.K. that they changed their minds. But the tone of the statement is off-key and the content does not address the clients' problems with her. By this point in the session it should be clear that the transferential issue needed to be faced.

Comments

C has a difficult task ahead of her because on one hand the clients have made an autonomous decision (and thus one goal of genetic counseling has been achieved), yet they feel defensive for having done so, as if they have let her down. How can she inhibit these transferential reactions, reduce their possible guilt feelings and defensiveness and achieve the nondirective goals of bolstering their autonomy and self-directedness? Her two well-meaning interventions seem to just miss the mark and, if anything, tend to increase the couple's need to justify themselves.

Perhaps at this point in the professional's career, her counseling skills have not matured and so she has difficulties achieving what she intends to accomplish. Also, she may not have a clear picture of her psychological goal and this may interfere with the words and tone she chooses to use at a given moment. Also, C may have begun the session with an agenda focused on reinforcing previously given information and may have been caught off-guard by the clients' agenda. From M's first words it become clear that this session may require counseling based on a model that is more psychologically oriented rather than information oriented.

Let us take a deeper look at this situation, keeping in mind that the goal of nondirective counseling is to promote the autonomy and self-directedness of the client (Kessler, 1997b). Two adults come to you and tell you that following previous counseling they have autonomously decided to proceed along a particular path. However, they seem to feel "guilty" toward you, as if they have disappointed you, and they seem to be defensive. Your inner dialogue might be something like the following:

> "What is going on here and how can I help them feel good about their decision, competent, and so on? I might not have made the same decision they did, but right now, my feelings are not relevant, so off to the mental back burner they go. Let me concentrate on them and let me first decide what's going on now."

The clue to what is going on, as the professional realizes, is contained in the phrase, "We both feel like guilty children. . . ." The relevant key word is children since this seems to be an apt description both of how they feel and are behaving toward the professional.

The professional might continue her inner dialogue as follows:

I wonder why they feel like children toward me? Perhaps they are projecting something concerning a past relationship on me. Is M making me into his mother? Perhaps something out of his past history, some possible act of disobedience, is being connected to the current situation and with the relationship with me. This might account for this guilty children business. They see me as parental and themselves as rebellious. Thus, even though they made an autonomous decision they don't feel good about it and can't take pride in it because it isn't coming from a place of autonomy, it's coming from a place of rebellion. This is transference we're talking about.

The professional has now identified the problem that needs attention and some of the psychodynamics that might be in play. The inner dialogue continues:

They're saying that they are disobeying me. But, that means they believe that I told them how to behave in the previous session and I didn't. I didn't give them any advice or suggestions they should use amniocentesis. So it's all their projection and I can say something to that effect to them.

But, wait. That's only my defensive voice speaking. If I said to them that I never advised them to have an amnio, would that contribute to their self-esteem and their feelings of competence? Probably not. On the contrary. It's likely to make them feel foolish for having their feelings; it might make them feel embarrassed; it might make them argumentative. All of that would not be helpful to them (or me). Also, my perception of what happened is less important than their perception. You know what they say, "The customer is always right." So, let's assume that they are right. Maybe unwittingly I told them what they should do. Maybe, I did imply or tell them, without realizing it, that they had to have an amnio. Wouldn't that account for their feelings? Yes, it would. Perhaps then it was I; I did or said something that undermined their autonomy and if I did that, intentionally or not, then perhaps I owe them an apology, because even though I didn't mean to "harm" them, perhaps I did.

This inner dialogue is an essential process of what many professionals go through in order to clarify to themselves what clients are saying and what they need to do and say to help them feel more in control, self-directed, and autonomous. This discourse remains private; it is rarely verbalized. It might lead to the following intervention:

C: Wait up! You don't owe me any explanation or rationale. If anything, I may owe you an apology for implying that you should or must have an amniocentesis when we met last year. That wasn't my intention; I just wanted you to know that if you decided you wanted an amniocentesis, it was available. But, maybe I was pushing amniocentesis too much back then or maybe I just wasn't making myself clear enough and I'm sorry I left you with the impression that you had to have the procedure. I sometimes get rather exuberant and possibly did try to oversell the procedure to you and I'm sorry about that. You're both two intelligent, competent grown-ups and you know what's best for your needs—certainly you know better about those things than I do—and obviously after giving yourselves time to think about it, you decided amniocentesis wasn't necessary. So I can respect your decision and no justification to me is necessary. So, how do you feel about having a baby?

EXAMPLE 3   **93**

What is the strategy here? First, the professional interrupts the justifications and bluntly states, "It's not necessary." This interferes with the clients' defensive process and shifts their full attention to what C is about to say next. Then she assumes responsibility for their need to justify themselves and offers an apology (as if to say, "It's my mistake, not yours. If I wasn't so incompetent or clumsy, you wouldn't need to sit here and justify yourselves now"). This is a key nondirective strategy that tends to accomplish multiple goals. It affirms the clients' reality, which tells them that they are not to blame for any misunderstandings between themselves and the professional. It also bolsters their sense of competence, relieves them of their defensiveness, and it tells them how fallible the professional is. In other words, in order to help the clients regain a sense of equal status with the professional, the latter deliberately reduces her own apparent status by pointing out how imperfect she has been (or is). This helps them establish a more mutual relationship with her rather than an unequal, parent–child one. She undercuts their childlike relationship to her and bolsters their adult sides by underscoring that they are intelligent adults and able to make their own decisions. Note she does not say that she supports their decision (she may not); since this would re-establish her status as an authority and reinforce the clients' sense of being children. She says she can respect their act of autonomy.

EXAMPLE 3

In this excerpt[4] (which was broadcast on CBS *Sunday Morning*) a woman has taken the predictive test for Huntington disease (HD) and is about to receive her results. Present are a male medical geneticist (G), a female counselor (C), the woman (W), and her husband (M).

1. C: I'm sorry [*unclear; perhaps: for keeping you waiting.*]
2. W: Oh, that's O.K.
3. G: I want to explain to you what's happened to the blood
4. test since you were last here. Essentially the blood was
5. assessed and the DNA changes have in fact indicated that you
6. have a CAG size that is in the range for somebody who will
7. develop Huntington disease at some time in the future.
8. C: Not exactly the news you were hoping to hear, huh?
9. W: [*subdued*] No.
10. C: But it's O.K. It's over with.
11. W: [*subdued*] Yeah.
12. G: It's not what we wanted to tell you today.
13. W: I know.
14. C: What does it feel like? Do you have a shock?

[4]Courtesy of CBS Current Affairs Program, *Sunday Morning*.

15. W: [*softly*] Sore.
16. M: [*softly*] Sore, yeah.
17. G: It is sore. The family, in the future and . . . [*breaks off*]
18. Where does it feel sore for you, in what areas?
19. W: [*unclear; possibly, In your chest.*]
20. C: How about you, T?
21. M: The same.

Summary

The session begins with an apology (1) that is handled graciously by W (2). G then explains that W is a likely gene carrier for HD. C enters the discussion immediately (8), presumably to make contact with W who seems crushed by the news (9) and confirms that she is disappointed by the results. C attempts to convey her caring (10) but W's response is one of numbness (11). G expresses his caring as if to apologize for being the bearer of bad news (12). Again, W acts graciously and accepts G's "apology" (13) in a way similar to what she did at (2). C asks W how she feels (14) and provides her own answer. W replies, "Sore" (15). G attempts to provide solace but breaks off when he realizes that he probably doesn't understand what W meant and he shifts to explore this issue. Both M and W remain almost monosyllabic for the rest of the excerpt.

Analysis

From the onset W sounds like a well-socialized, well brought up individual; she has social grace and knows the proper things to say and is probably fairly verbal. The "news" she receives has a tremendous impact and she is left virtually speechless. Thus, her response at (15) it is all the more conspicuous. She might have said that she felt *awful* or *disappointed* or *hurt* and any of these terms would have been understandable and would have gone by unnoticed. But *sore* stands out because it is unusual word and has multiple meanings. On one hand, it might mean sensitive or tender due to some ongoing wound or bruise, and on the other hand, it refers to being provoked, offended, irritated, and angry. The word may have been aptly chosen, because it is likely W intended both meanings. I suspect G realized (17, 18) that a double entendre was intended and changed his mind in midstream in order to probe W's possible dissatisfaction, etc.

There are other striking things about this brief interaction, which lasts a total of about 60 seconds. First, the interaction between G and W (12, 13) is an especially poignant moment of human contact and understanding between the two. The quality of this interaction is what all of us try to aim for in our professional work.

Second, the results of the testing are given within the first 23 seconds of the session. Thus, in a little over a half of a minute following the giving of such news, the clients are asked four or five somewhat difficult questions (8, 14, 18, 20). It is clear from their responses that these usually articulate individuals are not in any position to

EXAMPLE 3   **95**

deal with them. Too much is probably being demanded of them in too short a period of time. Also, by questioning them in this intense way, it tends to interfere with their emotional processing of the information and dampens out emotional expression. It is clear by (9) that this particular couple probably needed more time, perhaps even to be by themselves for a few minutes, to let their feelings out and allow them to commiserate and comfort one another.

Comments

The scenario is a familiar one to many professionals; they come bearing "bad" news and the usual discomfort in doing so is present. Anyone who has been in G's position would appreciate that no matter how such information is conveyed it never feels right. However, in his own way, he does his best to cushion the blow. For example, he does not say, "We found that you have the HD gene," rather he phrases it ("[Y]ou have a CAG size . . . in the range for somebody who will develop [HD] at some time in the future") in a way that requires W to draw the inference that *she* is one of those *somebodys*. In making her make that extra cognitive step, G has cushioned the impact of what he has said. This is a helpful strategy for many clients.

After the "news" is delivered G sounds gentle (12) and empathic and attempts to say something (17) to help them find meaning in their situation, which, as I pointed out above is abruptly broken off. It is unclear whether or not W's answer (19) is what G might have been looking for. W may be too well bred to express her anger, even at this point.

C's (8, 10) interactions are problematic. The statement at (8) reflects her perception of W's reaction to the news. It is neither empathic nor unempathic; it merely describes the reaction as she sees it. Coming on the heels of what G has just said, it feels intrusive and barely gives the clients a chance to catch their breath. She then tries to console W (10), however, what she says is not in touch with the reality of the situation since for the clients it is neither "O.K." nor is it "over" in terms of the problems they will have to face in the short- and long-term. I can only speculate that C's behavior is either shaped by inexperience, anxiety, or both. This may account for the questions (14) the answers to which are all too obvious. If W is irritated or angry (note the statement, "In your chest." (19)), she may have good reason.

What might C have done in this session? Strange to say, she might have been more effective had she remained silent, at least at this point in the interview, and simply acted as a supportive physical presence for the clients and for G. The latter had conveyed the news and seemed to be handling the situation more than adequately.

In the face of another person's emotional pain, silence is often a golden strategy. In more than one instance, after giving some couples the results of predictive testing, I quietly got up and said perhaps they needed a few moments to be alone. My intuition told me that for these couples (not all, mind you) my presence was inhibiting the expression of their tears. I tiptoed out of the room and could hear their sobs through the closed door. I spent a few minutes making them each a cup of tea and returned to the room and offered the tea to them. I then asked them if they were able to talk and when they said yes we talked only about practical issues, such as what they planned to do the rest of the day after they left the medical center (or my office), who, how, and when they planned to tell others about the results, how to handle and what to say to their children, and other instrumental issues. Feelings were the least important issue on which to focus at this time.

DISCUSSION

Until recently genetic counseling has dealt with parents of children conceived or born with a genetic disorder; most frequently, the clients were the parents. The goal of such counseling was to communicate information so that clients might make informed decisions about a current or forthcoming pregnancy and, in some cases, deal with psychosocial problems. Current genetic technology has made it increasingly possible to conduct counseling with the person directly impacted by the genetic information.

Although the genetic, psychological, and social situations arising in genetic counseling were never totally simple or straightforward, relatively speaking, the problems encountered in the genetic testing of Huntington disease, breast, ovarian and other cancers, Alzheimer's disease, the mental disorders, and the like are far more intricate. The genetic information is more complex and less understandable to professionals and laypersons alike and the implications of the information is sometimes unclear even to geneticists. Furthermore, the psychological context of such counseling is one in which the threat to the client's personal health, quality of life, and survivability is intensified to the point where, unless skillful counseling procedures are employed, not only is communication likely to be ineffective but the potential for inflicting psychological harm increases.

It may no longer be possible to simply use the teaching model of genetic counseling (Kessler, 1997a) that worked in past decades; greater attention may need to be paid to psychological dynamics and counseling skills. In addition, many of the same problems encountered by counselors in other fields—issues of transference, countertransference, dependency, among others—are likely to manifest themselves and may need special attention since these have been largely ignored in the training of genetic counselors.

It is becoming increasingly apparent that technology is changing so rapidly genetic counselors and other professionals can hardly keep up. Moreover, the demands of the genetic services of tomorrow are being faced with yesterday's ideas and concepts of the genetic counselor's role and functions. Genetic counselors of the 21st century may need far greater flexibility and counseling skill than those of today. In this regard it has become imperative to understand where and how genetic counselors succeed and fail, their strengths and limitations, so that the quality of counseling and communication might be improved. Publishing transcripts or even fragments of genetic counseling sessions is an important step in accomplishing these tasks. Reading them, I find, helps practitioners gain insights into their work and challenges them to ask themselves, How would I deal with this problem? What would I say at this point? Why? What would be my goal? This process can only lead to an overall improvement of skills.

In the examples above each professional showed a differing set of difficulties. The professional in the first example seemed to have difficulty in adopting a counseling stance, applying counseling skills, and controlling her countertransferential issues. Her approach emphasized her authority and, relative to C, her synoptic wisdom. She had a clear view of her own values and the zeal to promote them regardless of their impact on C, her mate, and possibly others. The overriding necessity to push C toward a termination of the pregnancy suggested a major lack of impartiality on P's part that may have blinded her to consider that her approach contained aspects of deception, one of the hallmarks of directive counseling.

P presented herself as an ally to C and may sincerely have believed that what she was doing was in C's best interest. But she failed to ascertain what C's interests were. Her strategy did not include the elucidation of C's thinking about what a child with Down syndrome might mean for her (and her absent husband). In other words, P gave advice and shared personal thoughts with little if any understanding of her client and her needs. A simple question might have opened to a discussion of all the issues P eventually touched on. Instead, P's strategy consisted of asking apparently innocuous questions that seemed to have two purposes: to undermine C's autonomy and to allow P an opportunity to urge her to have an abortion. These counseling difficulties might be thought of either in terms of an inflexible professional agenda, countertransference, or both.

The professional in the second example had considerable self-assurance and some experience. She had a problem adjusting her style to match that of the clients; this is a problem more of shade than of substance. For example, what she said, "if we discuss something a year ago . . . you're supposed to stick by that" (17–19), is said with a tone of sarcasm rather than of acceptance. Although it is intended to convey an empathic understanding, it does not do so because the tone is off-putting. The clients were already on the defensive and needed a less acerbic approach on the counselor's part. Also, she had difficulty developing a more comprehensive model of working that accommodated such psychological issues as transference. Associated with such a model is the need to reduce the clinical detachment the counselor tends to use so as to narrow the working distance to the clients.

The problems displayed by the professional in the last excerpt seem largely those of inexperience and require some closer examination not only by counselors but also by their teachers and supervisors and will be discussed in greater detail in a subsequent publication (Kessler, 2000). She was obviously trying her best, but she seemed ill-prepared to handle the emotionally intense situation she had to confront. It was like someone had pushed her into the deep end of the pool without first giving instructions on how to swim or float.

The professionals in the first two examples both showed difficulty in developing a good working-distance[5] with their respective clients. Both tended to be too removed, as if to emphasize their professional status or authority in relation to the clients. In the first example this interfered with the professional's ability to understand the client or to express empathy. In the second example, the professional seemed to adopt an

[5]By working distance I refer to the psychological, not the physical, space between professional and client.

informal tone in her work and yet she was so removed she could not see that her own behavior was the source of the clients' difficulties.

The problem of the latter professional is likely to be a recurrent theme in genetic counseling sessions of the future. The possible need for multiple sessions or overly lengthy ones (see, for example, Schneider, 1994; Peters and Stopfer, 1996) may make transferential phenomena more conspicuous. Similarly, the potential for the professional's personal involvement in the disease for which counseling is sought may increase countertransferential responses and may interfere with efforts to be neutral and to keep the clients' interests in the forefront. Any model of genetic counseling that tends to ignore or minimize psychological phenomena will be poorly equipped to handle the issues of transference and countertransference.

REFERENCES

Kelly PT (1977) Dealing with Dilemma. New York: Springer-Verlag.

Kessler S (1979) The genetic counseling session. In: Kessler S (ed.). Genetic Counseling: Psychological Dimensions. New York: Academic Press, pp 65–105.

Kessler S (1981) Psychological aspects of genetic counseling. Am J Med Genet 8:137–153.

Kessler S (1997a) Psychological aspects of genetic counseling. IX. Teaching and counseling. J Genet Counsel 6:287–296.

Kessler S (1997b) Psychological aspects of genetic counseling. XI. Nondirectiveness revisited. Am J Med Genet 72:164–171.

Kessler S (1997c) Transcripts of genetic counseling sessions: exercises in missed opportunities. Paper presented at Workshop, Talking Human Genetics: Verbal Communication, Knowledge and Genetic Make-up. April 24–27, 1997, Hamburg, Germany.

Kessler S, Jacopini AG (1982) Psychological aspects of genetic counseling. II. Quantitative analysis of a transcript of a genetic counseling session. Am J Med Genet 12:421–435.

Kessler S (2000) Emotional rescue [letter to the Editor] J Genet Counsel 9:275–278.

Michie S, Bron F, Bobrow M, Marteau TM (1997) Nondirectiveness in genetic counseling: an empirical study. Am J Hum Genet 60:40–47.

Peters JA, Stopfer JE (1996) Role of the genetic counselor in familial cancer. Oncology 159–166.

Schneider KA (1994) Counseling About Cancer: Strategies for Genetic Counselors. Boston, MA: Katherine A Schneider, MPH.

White MT (1997) "Respect for Autonomy" in genetic counseling: an anlysis and a proposal. J Genet Counsel 6:297–314.

8

Empathy and Decency[1]

Personal counseling is concerned with three related tasks: understanding the client, communicating that understanding, and, whenever possible, helping clients feel better about themselves or their circumstances. The initial tasks, as they relate to genetic counseling, were the focus of several previous publications (Kessler, 1997a, 1997b, 1997c; 1998). This paper discusses how genetic counselors might empower their clients to deal more effectively with their issues and feel better about themselves.

People can be empowered or helped to feel better in many ways. For example, education imparts knowledge that, in turn, helps a person feel more effective in certain circumstances (e.g., school, reproductive decisions). Education might also provide a basis for autonomous decision making. This implies that the person's self-evaluation might be raised when they perceive themselves as efficacious in making such decisions. Competent counseling might also maintain or raise the person's self-esteem and help them feel more effective. Among other things, counseling may assist people. The counselor must never make decisions for the (client) regarding marriage, children, and other important personal issues. These decisions are the (client's) responsibility and only (the client) should exercise this right to better understand their actions and decisions, to gain perspective, and to cope more effectively with their circumstances. In genetic counseling, professionals have an opportunity to use the techniques of both education and counseling to help their clients. However, the organization of genetic services and the pressures to provide complex information to clients tend to skew counseling practice in the direction of educational approaches (Kessler, 1997a). Thus, insufficient attention may be given to psychological issues

[1]This essay first appeared as Kessler S (1999) Psychological aspects of genetic counseling. XIII. Empathy and decency. *Journal of Genetic Counseling* 8:333–344. Reprinted with kind permission of the publisher, Kluwer Academic/Human Sciences Press.

and the psychological or counseling methods of dealing with such issues; a long-standing problem in the field (Reed, 1974; Sorenson, 1974; Antley, 1976; Falek, 1977; Kessler, 1979; Sorenson et al., 1981; Weiss, 1981; Schild and Black, 1984; Reif and Baitsch, 1985; Wertz et al., 1988; Shiloh and Saxe, 1989; Michie and Marteau, 1996).

Because of the magnitude of the dilemmas individuals and couples face when confronted with genetic risk, education alone may not provide an adequate basis for action or decision making. I may know that this object in front of me is a piano and I can be taught where to locate middle C on the keyboard, but that is a long way off from being able to play the Waldstein Sonata or, for that matter, "Chopsticks." Similarly, teaching clients about heredity and talking about models of coping or grieving are at some distance from translating concepts and ideas into practical everyday behavior. Furthermore, to cope effectively people need to have requisite coping skills. Without them, the educational process has the potential for promoting frustration, failure, and diminished self-esteem. Telling a student without study skills, for example, that they need to study harder is a recipe for drop-out behavior and negative self-evaluation. What needs to be learned is how to study. This might include learning to persevere, to anticipate and deal with inevitable pitfalls, and to mobilize other skills. Reversing maladaptive behavior requires attention to the assessment of what difficulties need to be overcome as well as what needs to be learned. In joining together educational and counseling procedures, meeting clients' needs is likely to be maximized.

EMPOWERING CLIENTS

In genetic counseling we supply complex facts and attempt to point clients in the right direction so that they see the goal ahead. But this may not be enough if they do not experience themselves as having—or do not have—the wherewithal to get there. This has the potential for personal failure. Take a simple example:

Example 1

A client is told that other siblings in her family may carry a certain gene and that it might be advisable to encourage them to be tested. The client is agreeable but her relationship with her sibs is so filled with conflict, even a short telephone conversation with them would be very difficult, perhaps aversive. She is embarrassed about the situation and about her own feelings and negative self-judgments, for example, her lack of "backbone," and it is likely she will not volunteer this shame-laden information to the professional. She assures the professional that she will take care of things right away and leaves the latter's office feeling somewhat depressed.

A genetic counselor who sees their role primarily as an educator might not probe to ascertain whether or not the client is able to follow through on the recommended behavior. This, unwittingly, might leave her feeling inadequate and possibly defeated and the chances of follow-through are low.

More directive professionals might take over the task of informing relatives themselves. Psychologically, this might increase the client's dependency on the former, undermine their autonomy, and reinforce their sense of inadequacy. Even for the best intentions directiveness may not always have positive consequences for clients.

Genetic counselors with a greater commitment to counseling strategies might feel obligated not only to ascertain the client's capability for follow-through but might help her deal with, and possibly overcome, the obstacles in the way of her feeling effective. For example, the counselor might reframe the blocks so that they do not have an aversive valence or might use skills training and rehearsal techniques (Meichenbaum and Fitzpatrick, 1993) in addition to encouragement and the provision of hope. In other words, a counseling professional would tend to be more active in providing the help the client needs to accomplish her particular goals, so that the outcome is more likely to be a sense of greater empowerment and enhanced self-esteem.

DECENCY

A major way of bolstering or buoying up the client's self-esteem is through simple decency. In practical terms, professionals need to express kindness, to raise the person's spirits, to give rewards, to bolster self-efficacy, and to teach and encourage the application of coping skills. All of these are core aspects of the counseling endeavor. In my view, no genetic counseling session, regardless of its length or content, should end without at least one sincere professional effort in this area. This might seem obvious, yet, surprisingly, it does not always happen. A not uncommon example of the latter situation follows.

Example 2

A woman came to a genetic counselor to discuss testing for the BRCA genes. She told the professional that she wanted to know her gene status so that she could prepare herself and her family for the future. She also informed the professional that she already had been diagnosed with breast cancer and had a mastectomy, an agonizing course of chemotherapy and radiation. In response to this information, the professional asked where the surgery and treatment were done, who did it, etc. and then moved on to discuss heredity and to provide risk figures. The session ended after information on testing was given.

Unwittingly the professional's response communicated several messages that, in sum, told the client that she could not expect much understanding from him. Thus an opportunity to express human interest and kindness was lost. She was treated as a case, not as a feeling human being; there was a lack of decency. In most instances this does not help clients to feel better about themselves or their situation. On the contrary, this professional's approach is likely to reinforce the woman's own feelings of being defective, unattractive, and unwanted.

What might have been a more effective counseling strategy? The professional might have tried to be more understanding. For example, he might have said something like,

"It sounds like you've been through a lot recently." Although this is a minimalist reflection of understanding, it is far superior to the detached approach above. If the professional truly needed the information on who did the surgery, etc., these questions might have been postponed and the opportunity to make greater human contact with the client given greater priority. If the professional had followed up the initial statement with further statements of understanding, as for example, "I wonder how you (your spouse, your kids, etc.) dealt with all that?" the client might likely have felt reassured that she was dealing with a professional with "a heart," someone really interested in her. This, in itself, has a salutory effect on the person, especially when they are struggling with issues of survival and self-image. When combined with positive reinforcements (see below) it has a powerful psychological potential.

THOUGHTFULNESS

The need for greater thoughtfulness in work with persons who have undergone major cancer surgery or treatment is imperative. The next example concerns a 36-year-old woman who has had a lumpectomy and completed a course of chemotherapy and radiation. She returned to her oncologist for a 6-month checkup and in an excited voice described how well she has been feeling (C = client; D = physician; N = nurse).

Example 3

C: Oh, and the kids are doing great and my husband's just got a promotion at work. And best of all, we just bought a new house in a great neighborhood and we're moving in 2 weeks. We're all so excited.

N: Oh, yes.

C: We just had to get out of the old house. It's too small and anyway I no longer have good feelings about it, you know. The cancer and everything.

N: Are you sure that's wise? You know the highest rate of recurrence of breast cancer happens in the first year.

C: [*bursts into tears*]

The physician enters the office. N leaves.

D: My, what's going on? You seem upset.

C: [*after composing herself*] I don't know. I came in today feeling so hopeful and excited for a change and Mildred [the nurse] told me, oh, I don't know [*begins to cry again*]. Maybe I'm being foolish. We've bought a new home and she said we were foolish to do so since my chances of a recurrence are so high.

D: Well, Mildred is right. The chances for recurrence are high in the first year. [*Risk figures are then discussed and the physician examines C and tells her things look all right.*]

This is a situation that occurs all too frequently in medical settings; the client's or patient's need for hope and support is undermined in a thoughtless way. This is not the setting to discuss what motivates some professionals to behave this way or what needs are gratified in doing so. Suffice it to say, these professionals were apparently not trained well in counseling practice. But, even with such training all of us know that, at some time, we have said thoughtless things to our friends, loved ones, clients, and others. Counselors know that they have a professional obligation to understand and control this tendency. A more thoughtful professional might have responded to the news about C's new home by either staying neutral (e.g., "Oh, that's interesting"), joining C in her excitement (e.g., "Oh how exciting!"), or by saying something empathic (e.g., "You want to make a fresh start after all you've been through.").

POSITIVE REINFORCEMENT

In taking a family or medical history counselors listen for data that can be reflected back to the client, at an appropriate time, as evidence of their accomplishments and strengths. These may be reminders that not everything in the client's life is negative. They might also be (simultaneously) positive reinforcements of ideas the clients have about themselves which validate their thinking or feelings. The following example illustrates this point (C = client; P = professional).

Example 4

C: About 3 years ago I had a stillborn child and became really depressed. I just wanted to die. I got into bed and didn't want to get up. After a while my doctor referred me to a psychiatrist who put me on Prozac and that's when I went into therapy. It was really helpful and I'm grateful for the help I got. In about 4 months or so I was doing much better and was even thinking about going back to school to finish my training as a dental hygienist. But it was about then my mother passed away and, as if that wasn't enough, I found out my husband was having an affair and that really did me in. We had a row, boy we did, and he walked out and I just wanted to, oh well, I finally divorced him last year.

P: What are you doing now?

C: Well, I did go back to my training and I'll be graduating next week, and I've got a job lined up with a dentist in my neighborhood.

P: So let me see if I understand. You had a stillborn child about 3 years ago and became depressed and needed treatment and anti-depressant medication. You went into therapy and apparently found it helpful. As you were coming back to yourself your mother died and you discovered your husband was having an affair. There were some heated moments and finally you divorced him a year ago. And despite all these setbacks you managed to go to school and fulfill what seemed to be a long-standing dream of yours to become a dental hygienist. And you've already got a job prospect. I bet you're proud of yourself!

Here the professional reflects back what he or she heard the client say. Note that the professional tries to feed back the material in the same order in which the client stated it, thus indicating that he or she was paying attention and taking the client seriously. Also note how the professional points out the client's accomplishments in spite of all her hardships, underscoring that they occurred as a consequence of her own efforts, not due to chance or the intervention of others. Clients often underestimate the effects of their efforts in making changes in their lives. When an outsider, especially one seen as an authority, points this out it tends to have a powerful impact.

CONSOLATION AND GIVING COMFORT

Some professionals may wonder, "How can I help a client feel better about their situation if I have to give them bad news?" Many may feel it is impossible to do so. But this is not necessarily true. In my experience, a simple, sincere word or two or even a touch may have an enormous impact on persons who have been devastated by calamity. Years afterwards, clients have reported how much something said by a counselor or a minister, priest, or rabbi had meant to them even though they were in the throes of suffering.

Example 5

I once had to give a woman the results of her testing for the Huntington disease (HD) gene; she carried a large expansion. She came to the session dressed casually and wearing a silver cross that she fingered during the information-giving portion of the session. Before the session was over I said to her that she needed to remember that the gene would affect only her body; her soul would remain functional and intact. This brought tears to her eyes and she whispered, "Thank you."

Small human touches like that often stay with the person long after the factual portions of sessions are forgotten and, in later recall, give solace and perspective to an individual's pain.

The following example is another instance in which an attempt to comfort a client is made despite the fact that devastating news is given.

Example 6

Mollie M. came into therapy with me (about 15 years ago) and I saw her for about five weekly sessions. She was at risk for HD but she seemed free of symptoms at that time. She had recently moved to the San Francisco Bay area and wanted to connect with a psychotherapist to deal with the stress of moving and her concerns about HD. In the sessions she inevitably talked about her past history. Her mother had died from HD and, as a child, she had been her major caregiver. She lived with her paternal grandparents for several years and they were important sources of emotional support. When they died she moved to the West Coast and in doing so broke off relations with her father and brother that were not very good to begin with. As a young adult she suffered a brain concussion and that left her with a tremor that she interpreted as a harbinger of HD symptoms. Presumably because of my age (and her need), she quickly developed a positive transference. In each session she would well up and cry and seemed surprised that that occurred. She could not identify what it was about our sessions that made her cry, but nevertheless seemed to experience a sense of relief in doing so. She told me that she had adopted a lesbian lifestyle and had found a group of women to live with.

Several years after we terminated therapy, I chanced to meet her in a bookstore, and I could see that she had become symptomatic with HD. We chatted briefly and I did not see her again for about 3 years, at which time she called me to say that she had undergone DNA testing for HD and that she wanted me to be with her at her current therapist's office when she obtained the results. After talking to the therapist I agreed to do so.

We met at the therapist's office and chatted briefly. She continued to live at a commune with her women friends, who seemed to take good care of her and provided strong emotional support. In the session the therapist handed me an envelope that contained the test results. I opened it and said, "I'm sorry to tell you but the results indicate that you have the HD gene." She began to cry and her therapist held her. We sat silently for a few moments and she reached out for my hand that I took and cupped into both of mine. Softly I began to speak: "I'm wondering Mollie, even though you might have wished that it would be different, I'm wondering if you hadn't expected that result when you took the test?" She nodded her head and whispered, "Yes." I waited a moment and said, "You were really brave then to go ahead with the testing." She did not reply and again we sat in silence as tears ran down her cheeks. At last she said, "I had to take it so that I could get on SSI [governmental disability payments] to cover the expenses of a wheelchair and all the other stuff I'm going to need in the future." "Yes, I understand," I said, "but it still took courage to do it," and again she nodded.

After a while I offered to show her the results and the three of us talked about them for about 10 minutes. Before I got up to leave I said, "You know Mollie you are such a wonderfully lovable person and people do care about you and love you. I can see that Janice [her therapist] cares a great deal about what happens to you and the women in the commune do too. And I care about you even though there isn't very much I can do to help you feel better about things except to be there for you when you need me. The things you described that they do for you in the commune they do out of love and caring and even though you have the cross of HD to bear, there are others there willing to help you carry the load. You are loved Mollie and that can't be said of everybody."

Which one of us does not want to hear someone they trust and respect tell them how good, how wonderful, how unique, lovable, generous, courageous they are? In our moments of pain and despair we have an especially desperate need to hear such words. They remind us of the qualities that, because of suffering, we ourselves cannot bring to mind. No professional deludes himself or herself into believing that such words will make a person instantly feel better about their awful situation. But, when pain eases, these words slowly filter into consciousness and re-awaken the person's soul and self-esteem. This is a sample of simple decency and kindness, something that can be made an integral part of every genetic counseling session.

DISCUSSION

Counselors strive to perfect their ability to understand clients, give them a sense of being understood, and help them feel more hopeful, more valued, and more capable of dealing with their life problems. Because genetic counselors work with people filled with uncertainty, fear of the future, anguish, and a sense of personal failure they have unusual opportunities to accomplish these tasks.

The samples of counseling behavior offered here hardly exhaust the many possible ways genetic counselors might ease their client's anguish and diminish their overall suffering. These strategies neither require much time nor complex skills. They merely give voice to the natural thoughtfulness and sensitivity we all have within us, characteristics that attracted us to the helping professions to begin with. Where counselors differ from most other professionals is that their mindset is geared to actively seek and create opportunities to express this aspect of themselves in their work.

The need for the greater application of counseling procedures in genetic counseling is likely to increase in the years ahead. First of all, clients will have increasing access to information off the Internet and may have a greater need for professional assistance in integrating it in their lives. Secondly, the "new genetics" increasingly confronts professionals with issues that tend to place them into the role of counselors or therapists rather than educators. The fact that the information they provide is emotionally evocative and intimately connected to the survival of the client requires counselors to make a deeper exploration of the personal meaning clients give to the information. Furthermore, such diseases as cancer cut close to home and often arouse countertransferential responses far different and more personally intense than those professionals had to face in the past. This may require professionals to engage increasingly in the inner "work" counselors and therapists need to do in order to work more effectively with clients. A professional woman in her thirties or forties talking to another woman of similar age who has been advised to have an oophorectomy or who has already lost a breast to cancer knows full well that tomorrow she might be the one seated in the client's chair. Lastly, inattention to the emotional meaning of information may become less acceptable to clients and professionals alike. A professional dealing with a person diagnosed with cancer who does not acknowledge their struggle for survival, as in Examples 2 and 3 above, is not only being unhelpful to the client, but may actually be inflicting psychological harm. Such clients need time to tell their stories, express their fears and pain, talk through their thoughts regarding treatment and related matters, and need a patient, sympathetic professional to provide them with a sense of hope and encouragement; the tasks of counseling.

Genetic counselors are increasingly finding that the traditional model of yesteryear may no longer apply to the problems raised by current genetic technology. The information has become more complex, the issues clients face more personal, decision making more uncertain, and psychological processing more complicated. The need for competent counseling has never been greater. In this regard, attention needs to be given to the factors believed to lead to successful outcomes in psychotherapy and other areas of personal counseling. These include what Seligman (1998) calls tactics of positive psychology such as paying attention to and developing rapport with clients and applying such procedures as instilling hope and courage, fostering interpersonal skills, emphasizing rationality and perseverance, and helping clients put problems in perspective so that they find meaning and purpose in their lives. All of these help build buffering capacities against the knocks of life, which, in turn, help clients deal more effectively with their problems. These counseling tactics and deeper strategies are certainly within the capacity of genetic counselors and, if they are not, can (and should) be acquired.

In my experience two arguments have been advanced to eschew the counseling aspects of genetic counseling: counseling would do harm and time constraints. One still hears assertions that counseling would "open up a can of worms" or "drag things out of people" or "leave them high and dry." In my opinion, such beliefs are irrational and are based on distorted ideas about human psychological needs and functioning. They tend to reflect the professional's anxieties and fears about human emotions and their feelings of inadequacy in counseling skills. Such inadequacies and anxieties are also too-often rationalized by suggesting that one is pressed for time and there is much information to convey. Indeed, genetic counselors are frequently under time constraints. However, as one reads transcripts of genetic counseling sessions (Kessler, 1999) one is impressed by how much time there actually is to give something to clients besides information. The paucity of process studies hinders us from finding ways to make the educational and counseling aspects of genetic counseling more effective.

The arguments against the counseling side of genetic counseling have been with us for far too long. They provide support for the maintenance of an unsatisfactory status quo that tends to frustrate the giving of greater psychological understanding and support to clients—there is no limit in this regard—and interferes with the honing of professionals' counseling skills. In time, it is my hope, that many professionals will experience this antipathic stance as being unworthy of their talents and human capacities.

REFERENCES

Antley RM (1976) Variables in the outcome of genetic counseling. Soc Biol 23:108–115.

Falek A (1977) Use of the coping process to achieve psychological homeostasis in genetic counseling. In: Lubs HA, de la Cruz F (eds). Genetic Counseling. New York: Raven Press, pp 179–188.

Kessler S (1979) The genetic counselor as psychotherapist. Birth Defects: Original Article Series 15(2):187–200.

Kessler S (1997a) Psychological aspects of genetic counseling. IX. Teaching and counseling. J Genet Counsel 6:287–295.

Kessler S (1997b) Psychological aspects of genetic counseling. X. Advanced counseling techniques. J Genet Counsel 6:379–392.

Kessler S (1997c) Psychological aspects of genetic counseling. XI. Nondirectiveness revisited. Am J Med Genet 72:164–171.

Kessler S (1998) Psychological aspects of genetic counseling. XII. More on counseling skills. J Genet Counsel 7:263–278.

Kessler S (2000) Reading transcripts: missed opportunities in genetic counseling. In: Hartog J, Wolff G (eds). Talking Human Genetics: Verbal Communication, Knowledge and Genetic Make-up (in preparation).

Meichenbaum D, Fitzpatrick D (1993) A constructivist narrative perspective on stress and coping: stress inoculation applications. In: Goldberger L, Breznitz S (eds). Handbook of Stress. New York: Free Press.

Michie S, Marteau T (1996) Genetic counseling: some issues of theory and practice. In: Marteau T, Richards M (eds). The Troubled Helix: Social and Psychological Implications of the New Human Genetics. Cambridge: Cambridge University Press, pp 104–122.

Reed S (1974) A short history of genetic counseling. Soc Biol 21:332–339.

Reif M, Baitsch H (1985) Psychological issues in genetic counselling. Hum Genet 70:193–199.

Schild S, Black RB (1984) Social Work and Genetics. New York: Haworth Press.

Seligman MEP (1998) Why therapy works. APA Monitor 29:2.

Shiloh S, Saxe L (1989) Perception of risk in genetic counseling. Psychol Hlth 3:45–61.

Sorenson JR (1974) Genetic counseling: some psychological considerations. In: Lipkin M Jr, Rowley PT (eds). Genetic Responsibility. New York: Plenum Press, pp 61–67.

Sorenson JR, Swazey JP, Scotch NA (1981) Reproductive Pasts, Reproductive Futures: Genetic Counseling and its Effectiveness. Birth Defects Original Article Series 17(4):1–192.

Weiss JO (1981) Psychosocial stress in genetic disorders: a guide for social workers. Soc Work Health Care 6:17–31.

Wertz DC, Sorenson JR, Heeren TC (1988) Communication in health professional-lay encounters: how often does each party know what the other wants to discuss. In: Ruben BD (ed). Information and Behavior, Vol 2. New Brunswick, NJ: Transaction, pp 329–342.

9

A Critical Review of the Literature Dealing with Education and Reproduction[1]

INTRODUCTION

Most of the past relevant research involving psychological variables is concerned with effects or effectiveness of genetic counseling. Because for many counselors genetic counseling is primarily an educational activity, numerous studies have been conducted in which the memory for diagnostic or recurrence risk information has been evaluated. For some counselors genetic counseling is seen as a means of reducing the incidence of genetic disease in human populations, and thus, there also has been a strong interest in determining the effectiveness of counseling in altering reproductive intentions or behavior. Hsia (1977), Shaw (1977), Childs (1978), and Evers-Kiebooms and van den Berghe (1979) reviewed the literature before 1979.

In their assessment of the literature, Evers-Kiebooms and van den Berghe (1979) argued that no strong conclusions about the impact of genetic counseling could be drawn. Results of investigations on the understanding of genetics and memory for recurrence risks varied widely from study to study, and largely because of their retrospective designs, it was not possible to determine whether or not the counseling had been adequate or effective. Also, in evaluating reproductive plans or behavior following genetic counseling, it was not clear that the decisions made by counselees resulted from or were influenced by the counseling.

The decade following their review continued to be active in terms of research on genetic counseling and this current literature is reviewed here. Since methodological problems tended to persist, more than usual attention will be given to the materials

[1]This essay first appeared as Kessler S (1989) Psychological aspects of genetic counseling. VI. A critical review of the literature dealing with education and reproduction. *American Journal of Medical Genetics* 34:340–353. Reprinted with kind permission of the publisher, John Wiley and Sons.

and methods of the individual studies under review. The present focus is less on the effectiveness of genetic counseling per se (this cannot entirely be ignored) than on an examination of how psychological variables have been studied and what light such investigations shed on the process of genetic counseling. Following an introductory statement, the studies to be reviewed will be grouped under two general topic headings:

1. Education
   a. Outcome studies
   b. Process studies
2. Reproduction
   a. Outcome studies
   b. Process studies

In a subsequent publication the topic of risk perception and interpretation will be considered.

The research will be examined generally in chronological order. The few studies of such psychological issues as self-concept, guilt, anxiety, mood, and similar concepts will not be evaluated here since these generally involve unstable measures of situation-specific or population-specific responses. Generalities outside the specific study should be drawn cautiously. Also, a handful of studies dealing with client satisfaction with genetic counseling will not be considered as part of this review since none of these have provided controls for socially desirable responses.

The reader is cautioned that many of the studies are difficult to assess and to compare. Different investigators may have focused on different genetic disorders, some with high recurrence risks and others with low or negligible ones, some for which prenatal diagnosis is available and others where it is not possible. Also, in some studies gaps in the description of materials and methods have occurred that make the total comprehension of results difficult. In some of the studies it is not always clear whether a given population number refers to an individual, a couple, or a family. Where families rather than individuals are reported, it is frequently ambiguous whether or not all relatives were included or if the data are based on the opinions and viewpoints of a single spokesperson. The amount of time elapsing between the counseling and the initiation of the study is often unclear. Data gathering in some investigations occurs over a relatively long period of time, whereas in other studies this period may be relatively short. The results of the former studies may be contaminated by secular trends and by changes in genetic technology, counseling, or research personnel, etc. How some investigators gather data is ambiguous. The format and wording of questions in questionnaires are frequently not provided in the published report and, at times, insufficient attention has been given to item construction. Scales for measuring attitudes or perceptions sometimes seem arbitrary and, in some questionnaires, scoring problems are apparent. The quality of data presentation or analysis also leaves much to be desired. In some studies, groups are combined for analysis in ways that do not always lead to clarity or allow the curious reader to do his or her own analysis of the data. Information about the counselors, their training and orientation, is frequently missing and how the counseling was provided is frequently inadequately described. Several investigators have reported that counseling was nondirective. However, none have defined exactly what they meant by nondirectiveness.

In wrestling with the literature below, the reviewer has sometimes written to or discussed a study with the original investigators to obtain greater clarity on fine points. In most cases, investigators were forthcoming and cooperative. In a few instances, original data were provided or the reviewer recalculated results from the published report. If errors occurred as a consequence of such calculations or misinterpretations of the data were made, the reviewer takes full responsibility for them.

REVIEW OF LITERATURE

Education

Most past research in this area of genetic counseling tends to focus on either *recall* of information, as, for example, asking a person in an interview what diagnosis was given to his or her child, or the *recognition* of information as, for example, identifying on a multiple choice questionnaire the correct risk a person obtained in counseling. Recall and recognition memory involve distinct, yet interrelated, cognitive processes, and it is not clear whether studies calling for these differing memory functions are comparable.

Early evaluation studies have often assumed that recurrence risks and diagnostic information needed to be remembered accurately for decision-making purposes. The success of genetic counseling was measured by the extent to which accurate recall or recognition of these variables occurred following counseling. Investigators also tended to assume that the process of education in genetic counseling involved the *transfer* of information from counselor to counselee. Information transfer implied that the counselee received information passively in the same form and quality in which it originated. Also, it was assumed that human memory functioned like a tape recorder, reproducing information exactly as it was stored. When research found that distortion and inaccuracies in recall occurred, these were often attributed to the counselees' lack of pertinent education or to psychological defensiveness. Suggestions that counselors or their educational methods were inadequate were rare.

Unquestionably, many counselees come to genetic counseling to obtain information, particularly concerning genetic risk, etiology, and diagnostic issues (Sorenson et al., 1981) and such information is frequently used to make decisions about reproduction and other important life decisions (e.g., where to live so as to be near medical facilities, who to marry, etc.). However, it is doubtful that the information obtained in counseling is used in decision making exactly in the form in which it is acquired. To be useful for decision making, information first needs to be coded and stored in ways in which it can be accessed for later problem solving. To be coded and stored, information has to be transformed into personally meaningful units, which interface and, to greater or lesser extent, integrate with previously stored information. It is the *personal meaning* of information and not objective details which is stored and made available for later problem solving and decision making.

Outcome Studies

Black (1979) conducted an in-home interview study of parents of children with Down syndrome (DS) or with mental retardation of unknown causes (UK). At the time of the study, the children were 7 years old or younger; the average age of the parents in the DS group was 35 years and in the UK group it was 31 years. The groups were otherwise matched on the basis of education, income, years married, and number of children, although the UK parents tended to have more severely affected children and, because of their age, smaller families and less experience with a normal child. The DS group consisted of 11 couples and 5 single parents, and the UK group consisted of 10 couples. All had received genetic counseling and interviews of each parent separately occurred, on average, about 2.5 years after the counseling.

Black found that 73% of the DS and 55% of the UK parents were aware of having an increased recurrence risk. However, only 16% of the former parents, compared to 73% of the latter, had a correct recall of their respective risks. Among the DS parents, 32% could not recall a specific risk figure and 37% either over- or underestimated their risks. Among the UK parents, 18% could not recall a specific risk figure and 9% either over- or underestimated their risks. Black speculated that the better relative recall among the UK parents might have been due to the availability of prenatal diagnosis for DS; hence, DS parents did not need to recall their risks accurately or the risks had low salience for them. Also there was a possibility that the risk figure might have stood out as a solid fact for the UK parents in a counseling session that might have focused on the vague and uncertain cause of the retardation of their children.

Abramovsky et al. (1980) conducted a retrospective questionnaire study of 212 families who received genetic counseling during a 5-year period; it was emphasized that the counseling was nondirective. The questionnaire was said to consist of 31 multiple-choice questions covering a variety of subject areas including knowledge of risks, diagnosis and inheritance, reproductive intentions, and satisfaction with the counseling. Questions regarding diagnosis and recurrence risks were as follows:

"Was a specific diagnosis of the problem made or confirmed when you were seen in (the clinic)?"

"If yes, what was the diagnosis?"

"Were you given risk figures relating to your chances to have a child affected with the disease or condition?"

"What specific risk figures were you given?"

Closer examination of the other questions shows that nearly half of them required a yes or no answer and were not multiple-choice questions.

The data were compiled and pertinent answers were compared to information contained in medical records. Only one questionnaire was sent to each couple and it was not determined who actually completed the form. It was found that 91% of the couples recalled the specific diagnosis, 72% recalled the correct risk figures, and 56% were able to specify the correct mode of inheritance of the disorder on a multiple-choice question. The criteria used to determine "correctness" of recall were not given in the report and it cannot be assumed that "correct" recall of risks necessarily meant exact recall.

Seidenfeld and Antley (1981) studied 47 women who had a child with Down syndrome less than 1 year of age. All were counseled about 6 weeks after the diagnosis was made, at which time precounseling baseline information was gathered by questionnaires and interview. In the interview, the subjects were asked 13 questions regarding their knowledge about the genetics of Down syndrome, recurrence risks, and prenatal diagnosis. No information was given as to the criteria used to score answers as correct or incorrect.

For the total sample, the mean number of questions answered correctly before counseling was 6.2 and after counseling it was 10.6, a substantial increase. Only five of the subjects did not show a change in their scores. Examining specific areas of knowledge, it was found that of the three questions about general genetics, 26% of subjects could not answer any of the questions correctly, 64% could answer correctly one or two of the questions, and only 10% could answer all three questions correctly. After counseling, all subjects could answer at least one question correctly; 80% were able to answer all three questions correctly. In response to two questions about recurrence risks, 48% of subjects answered both correctly before counseling and 87% did so after counseling; 25% could answer neither question correctly before and 2% after counseling.

Broken down according to the subjects' educational level, those with less than a high school education showed the most improvement on their postcounseling scores, whereas those with more than a high school education showed the least gains. The authors suggest that the former group obtained about 70% of their knowledge from the counseling, whereas the latter subjects obtained only 27% of their knowledge from the counseling. This might be a scaling artifact since the latter group had a higher mean score than the former before counseling and there was a ceiling as to how high their scores could change.

Sorenson et al. (1981) conducted a prospective, longitudinal study of individuals and couples seeking genetic counseling in one of 47 clinics located in 25 states in the United States and the District of Columbia. Information was obtained largely by structured self-administered questionnaires given prior to counseling, approximately 1 to 2 weeks after counseling, and again 6 months later. The information included sociodemographic data, the reasons for seeking counseling, genetic knowledge and reproductive intentions before and after counseling, and a report of the content of the counseling session. The counselees were all seeking genetic counseling for the first time and had a command of the English language; most were married and between 20 and 34 years old. About 43% of the counselees had a living child with a birth defect or genetic disorder and 14% had an affected child who was deceased by the time they sought counseling; about 7% had sustained a miscarriage, 5% were pregnant for the first time, and 18% had never been pregnant. The 203 genetic counselors involved in the study, two-thirds of whom had medical degrees, also completed detailed questionnaires after the counseling session in which their perceptions were obtained.

To ascertain the counselee's knowledge of the diagnosis of the disorder or problem for which they were seeking counseling, they were asked to name and describe it. Their responses were then compared to those given by the genetic counselor after seeing the counselee. The accuracy of counselee responses was scored independently by two judges (reliability was over 90%). The investigators gave only data on female counselees. It was found that before counseling, 58% of the 1097 counselees in the study had an accurate knowledge of the diagnosis for which they were seeking genetic counseling and an additional 18% had a marginally accurate knowledge of the diagnosis; about 24% had an inaccurate knowledge, which included incorrect descriptions, such responses as "Did not know" or no responses, and (included here, since counseling had not yet occurred) a small number of cases listed as "No counselor diagnosis given." After counseling, omitting the cases for which no diagnosis was given, about 71% of counselees had an accurate and 17% a marginally accurate knowledge of the diagnosis and 13% had an inaccurate knowledge. There was a 17% increase in the accuracy category, but a 54% decrease in the number of counselees who had an inaccurate knowledge of the diagnosis. Looked at a different way, Sorenson et al. (1981) found that only 5% of the counselees who came to genetic counseling with an accurate or marginally accurate knowledge of diagnosis left counseling with an inaccurate knowledge, whereas of the counselees who came with an inaccurate knowledge of diagnosis, nearly 60% left with an accurate or marginally accurate knowledge. At the 6-month follow-up, about 10% of the group still had an inaccurate knowledge of the diagnosis. In sum, then, these data suggest that genetic counseling is effective in improving the counselees' knowledge of diagnostic information, especially when such information was inaccurate to begin with.

To ascertain the effects of genetic counseling on educating counselees about genetic risks, each counselee was asked to indicate the risk before, shortly after, and 6 months after genetic counseling. Before genetic counseling only 6% of 1097 counselees had an exactly accurate knowledge of the numeric risk for the problem for which they were seeking counseling. After counseling, 22% had an exactly accurate recall of the risk. Strict criteria, perhaps overly so, were used to define an accurate response. An accurate recall was scored as such only if the counselee was precise in giving the risk figure. If the cases for which no numeric risk was provided by the counselor are omitted from the analysis, the picture improves dramatically; 13% of counselees had an accurate knowledge of risk before counseling, but 51% had such knowledge after counseling, almost a 300% improvement. At the 6-month follow-up, 42% of the counselees remaining in the study who had been given a numeric risk had an accurate recall of the risk.

Examined as a function of accuracy or inaccuracy prior to and after counseling, the data show that 16% of counselees given a numeric risk who had an accurate idea of the risk before counseling left counseling with an inaccurate idea, whereas 46% of counselees who had an inaccurate idea of the risk before counseling had an accurate idea afterwards. These data are impressive in demonstrating that genetic counseling is effective in teaching counselees about genetic risks, particularly those who start off with less than accurate ideas. However, as Sorenson et al. (1981) point out, there is room for improvement, since about half of counselees who had an inaccurate idea of the genetic risk continued to have inaccurate ideas after genetic counseling.

The data of Sorenson et al. (1981) also suggest that over time the precise recall of risk decreases. This is not surprising given that there generally are no practice sessions to reinforce the initially acquired information or to mitigate against competing sources of information that might be consulted after genetic counseling was completed. Oetting and Steele (1982) carried out a questionnaire and interview study of 23 pairs of couples with a Down syndrome child; half the couples had received genetic counseling following the birth of the child and half had not. The former couples apparently had received counseling between 5 and 10 years before the start of the study. Otherwise the families were matched on the basis of race, religion, maternal age, paternal occupation, parental education, and sex and sibship order of the affected child. An interview was carried out on 11 pairs of couples and a test of general genetics knowledge was conducted. The latter test consisted of eight questions requiring the subjects to understand the principles of recessive inheritance, probability, and chromosomal sex determination and to be able to define a gene and a chromosome. However, the answer to one of the questions depended on giving a correct answer to the immediately preceding question and since the options for responses to three of the questions were yes and no, guessing might have been promoted. Also, it is unclear how the data were analyzed and how within-couple differences in responses, if and when they occurred, were handled statistically. In any case, these investigators reported no significant differences between the counseled and noncounseled couples in general genetic knowledge or in knowledge of the recurrence risk for Down syndrome. No strong conclusions can be drawn from these data.

Keltikangas-Jarvinen and Autio (1983) in Finland, studied 23 mothers, 20 fathers, and 34 siblings (gender unspecified) from 32 families with at least one member affected with aspartyglucosaminuria (AGU). Parents of affected children all had received verbal information about the disorder from their physicians and 1 year before the study began had also received a pamphlet in which the manifestations and course of the disorder was described as well as its genetics, pathogenesis, and methods of diagnosis and carrier detection. The time interval between initial diagnosis and the start of the study was 2–4 years. Although no supporting data were given, the families were said to be representative, socially and educationally, of Finnish AGU families. A structured interview was conducted in the home in which "simple" questions were posed based on the material in the pamphlet. In response to questions covering 10 topics, the best performance of parents involved a question on the mode of inheritance of the disorder; 17% of mothers and 35% of fathers answered correctly. On the topic of the meaning of recessive inheritance, 23% of sibs were able to answer this question correctly. Answers on all other questions ranged from 0% to 21% correct for all subjects. It turned out that only 34% of subjects had read the pamphlet and that, in spite of the poor recall of information, 80% of subjects expressed the view "that they knew all the essential aspects of the AGU disease and that they did not need any more information." The design of this study is flawed in several ways. Nonetheless, it illustrates how different the perceptions of providers and clients can sometimes be. One wonders what structural or other factors were present that contributed to the communicational chasm that seemed to exist in this particular setting.

Rowley et al. (1984) compared three different styles of genetic counseling—counseling provided by a trained physician (conventional counseling), videotaped counseling followed by an opportunity to question a trained physician (programmed counseling), and patient-structured counseling in which it was said that the content and affective tone of the counseling was "continuously modulated according to the verbal and nonverbal responses of the patient" (see below for materials and methods). The subjects consisted of persons detected in the course of screening and found to be beta-thalassemia trait carriers and matched controls who were negative for trait. Experimental subjects were randomly assigned to one of the three counseling methods. These investigators found no significant differences in knowledge of thalassemia and of genetics between 142 experimental and 123 control subjects prior to counseling. However, immediately after counseling and up to 10 months later, experimental subjects showed significantly greater acquisition and retention of information about thalassemia and genetics than did controls. Compared to the precounseling baseline scores, the mean knowledge scores of the experimental groups nearly doubled after counseling. There were no significant differences between the different styles of counseling on these measures.

Ekwo et al. (1985) studied pregnant women who were referred for amniocentesis for maternal age or a family history of Down syndrome. These investigators explored the subjects' objective and subjective assessments of risk for having a child with Down syndrome. The persons studied included 202 women who assented to the amniocentesis procedure and 50 women who declined the procedure. In the former group, 38% of the women for whom the age was available were 35 years old or younger; 35% were between ages 36 and 38; and 20% were 39 years of age or older. In the group declining amniocentesis, 30% if the women were 35 years of less in age; 42% were between ages 36 and 38; and 28% were 39 years or older; the age distribution seemed to be shifted upward (no means were given). The subjects were said to be predominantly middle or upper middle class. Interviewers who had 2–3 years of interviewing experience carried out a structured interview. For the group accepting amniocentesis, the interview was carried out after they received genetic counseling and consented to the procedure but before the procedure was done. For the group declining amniocentesis, the interview was carried out between the 18th and 22nd week of gestation. All subjects had been given standardized written information about their genetic risk. The objective risk was obtained by asking each subject to recall the specific risk given to her in genetic counseling. Data were obtained for 198 women who accepted amniocentesis and 49 of the women who declined the procedure.

In scoring the accuracy of the objective risks, the investigators accepted as accurate recall an age-appropriate risk figure ±1 year. Among the women who assented to the amniocentesis, 44% had an accurate recall of their risk, whereas among the group who declined the procedure only 29% had an accurate recall. Although Ekwo et al. (1985) found a positive correlation between education level and knowledge of the genetics of Down syndrome, there was no correlation between education level and the correct recall of objective risks. Strongly associated with the correct recall of objective risks for women who assented to the amniocentesis was their age; relatively older women were more likely than younger ones to recall risks correctly. Also, women who perceived the condition as relatively more burdensome tended to recall the objective risk more accurately than those who saw it as less burdensome. For women declining the procedure, the lower the parity and the poorer the knowledge of the genetics of Down syndrome, the less likely they were of recalling objective risks accurately; also when these individuals strongly believed that life must be saved at all costs, they were more likely to have an accurate recall.

These data might be explained by the greater salience risks had for the women who were to undergo the procedure as opposed to those who had declined the procedure. (This is exactly the opposite of the argument proposed by Black (1979) to explain her data.) Also, for women to believe that their risks were relatively high after they declined the amniocentesis procedure might create dissonance in their thought processes. They might think poorly of themselves or might feel others might judge them negatively if they thought their child was at high risk for a birth defect and they did nothing to prevent it. Ekwo et al. (1985) also found that the women who declined amniocentesis seemed more concerned about the possibility of being placed into a position where they might have to consider an abortion than women who accepted the procedure. Thus, by declining the amniocentesis they not only avoided having to face the issue of abortion, they also avoided the possibility of violating internal standards that might produce negative self-judgments.

Swerts (1987) conducted in-home interviews of 94 families who had a child with a neural tube defect. Among the latter families 47% had a child with anencephaly and 53% had a child with spina bifida. In all the families the maternal age at the birth of the child was 35 years or less and the child was either the first or second in the birth order. The families were divided into three groups: those who had received neither genetic counseling nor amniocentesis (n = 23), those who had genetic counseling but no amniocentesis (n = 29), and those who mostly (81%) had genetic counseling and amniocentesis (n = 42). The groups that were not counseled turned out to be less well educated than the counseled groups. It was not clear how long after counseling the interviews were conducted. About 3–6 years after the interview, families were recontacted by mail and asked to complete a questionnaire. Data were presented in terms of families rather than as individuals; thus within-couple disagreements of perception were ignored. Swerts remarked that 33% of the time, both partners were present for the interview and when a partner was absent they were asked to fill out and mail back a questionnaire.

Swerts found that 65% of the counseled parents and 29% of the uncounseled ones were able to recall the recurrence risk accurately. None among the former group and 10% among the latter one thought that they had no risk at all. About 23% of the counseled parents and 32% of the uncounseled ones could not recall any numeric risk. At the end of the interview, the parents were told the correct risk figure and pertinent literature was left. However, on the follow-up questionnaire it was found that 39% (n = 76) of all parents had an accurate recall of the risk figure whereas at the interview conducted closer to the initial counseling 56% of this group had an accurate recall of the risk. There was considerable decay over time of an accurate recall of risk despite the fact that written material was left with the families.

Swerts also ascertained the recall or knowledge of the incidence of neural tube defects in the general population and found that 46% of the counseled and 16% of the uncounseled group had an accurate knowledge. Among the counseled parents, 49% could not provide a numeric estimate whereas among the uncounseled group 74% could not provide an estimate. When asked to compare their risk for a child with a neural tube defect with that of parents who did not give birth to an affected child, 80% (n = 61) of the counseled group and 38% (n = 26) of the uncounseled group were aware that their risks were relatively higher. Swerts summarized her data as follows:

> The . . . data made it clear that the recall of the correct risk figures was substantially better in the counseled group than in the uncounseled group. A substantially large number of families, however, that [had genetic counseling] were found not to be aware of the correct recurrence and incidence figures. When the answers of the same parents on all knowledge-items were compared the degree of correct knowledge became even more disappointing. Only 17 out of the 63 . . . families that [were counseled] and one of the 31 families that did not receive genetic counseling answered all questions about risk figures . . . accurately. Even more striking was that a number of parents gave contradictory answers to the different questions such as being no longer at risk although knowing their correct . . . recurrence risk. Obviously, a number of parents "knew" risk figures but did not understand their meaning.

In another study described by Evers-Kiebooms et al. (1984), the sample consisted of 119 couples who had a child with Down syndrome; criteria to enter the study and description of methods are the same as in those of Swerts's 1987 study with the following differences. Only in 62% of the families were both parents present for the postcounseling interview and 80% of the couples responded to the follow-up questionnaire. As in the Swerts study, the educational level of the couples in the counseled group was higher than that of the uncounseled couples. Among the 76 couples who received genetic counseling, 45% recalled accurately the recurrence risk they obtained in counseling, 21% either over- or underestimated the risk, and 34% could not recall any numeric risk. Among the 43 couples who had not been counseled, 21% had an accurate knowledge of the risk, 26% had an inaccurate knowledge, and 54% could give no numeric risk figure.

Process Studies

Zorzi et al. (1980) studied 236 parents of 188 Down syndrome children in order to ascertain parental perceptions of the information and services they thought they needed in genetic counseling and the adequacy of the information and services they actually received. Parents were recruited through service agencies and voluntary organizational newsletters. Almost 91% of the parents were married at the time of the study and about 25% were planning to have more children. Questionnaires were mailed to some parents and distributed to others through local agencies as well as at support group meetings; the exact number of questionnaires distributed was unknown. Of the 188 questionnaires in the analysis, 69% were completed by the mother, 5% by the father, and 26% by both parents together. Only 55% of parents had actually received genetic counseling. In the questionnaire, parents were asked to rate, on a four-point scale, from most important to not important, each of 31 items thought to be pertinent to parents of a Down syndrome child. Also, parents were asked to respond yes or no on each item as to whether they had received adequate information during their own initial counseling experience.

The investigators found that, overall, 93% or more of parents thought it most important or important that they receive information on such topics as diagnosis, education, infant stimulation groups, medical care and special activities for the child, expectations as the child grows and prognosis, child's general care, relief of guilt, and how Down syndrome happens; these accounted for the 10 highest-ranked items. Recurrence risks (endorsed by 92% of parents) ranked number 11. Verbal information on genetics (86%) ranked number 15 and written information (80%) ranked number 17. Personal therapy (71%) and amniocentesis (66%) ranked numbers 19 and 20, respectively. The five lowest-ranked items were, in order of highest to lowest, institutions (34%), sexual therapy (32%), abortion (23%), foster care (21%), and sterilization (20%).

In response to the question, "Did you receive adequate information on this item?" at least 60% of parents (no total sample size given) of Down syndrome children 2 years of age or less were satisfied (i.e., they answered yes to the question) with 20 of 22 of the top-ranked items; at least 60% of parents with children between 3 and 5 years of age were satisfied with 17 out of the top 22 items; at least 60% of parents with children between age 6 and 12 were satisfied with 6 of the top 22 items; and less than 60% of parents with Down syndrome children 13 years of age or older were satisfied with any of the top 22 items. Thus, parents who reported receiving adequate information on most topics tended to have younger affected children. These parents also tended to have had genetic counseling.

Despite methodological flaws and, presumably, sampling biased toward parents of home-reared Down syndrome children who were also motivated to belong to voluntary organizations and to respond to the research questionnaire, this study suggests that information on recurrence risks and genetics may not be the top priority topics for such parents; pragmatic information on the care, education, prognosis, expectations of their children, and psychosocial support appear to be as important, if not more so, in the minds of these parents. The study also suggests that, although there is room for improvement in services, current informational services are more effective than past ones in filling client needs. The possibility that older parents may become dissatisfied over time with the information they received earlier cannot be ruled out since this variable was not controlled for in the study. Given the fact that not all of the subjects had received genetic counseling, the authors had an opportunity to compare counseled and uncounseled groups; if this was done, the data were not reported.

Whitten et al. (1981) described a program to provide sickle cell trait counseling and data on the educational performance of counselees and of counselors. The former were adults who had, or whose children had, sickle cell trait. Subjects were recruited through advertisement in the media and by other means. The counseling process required the counselor to adhere to a systematic format in which various pertinent topics were covered including a discussion of test results, a differentiation of sickle cell disease and trait, and a presentation regarding the reproductive options open to persons with trait and the reasons individuals or couples with trait do or do not have children. The counseling was provided by appropriately trained lay persons following a 15 minute slide-tape presentation that provided an overview of sickle cell disease and trait. At the beginning and again at the end of the counseling session the counselor asked the counselee, "How do you feel about having sickle cell trait?" or "How do you feel about your child having sickle cell trait?" Counseling sessions were audiotaped and during the course of the session the counselor asked 10 questions presumably shortly after the pertinent information was given to the counselee. The tapes were analyzed to determine how many of the questions were answered correctly. Also, the responses to the "feeling" questions were scored as either negative, positive, acceptance, or no feelings.

Expressions of anxiety, concern, or disavowal were scored negatively. Expressions of relief that it was only a trait were scored positively. Expressions like "It's just one of those things" were scored as acceptance. In the presentation of the results, expressions of acceptance were combined with the positive category. This is unfortunate since such responses could also be seen as evasions of the question and could have been combined with the "no feeling" category. It is unclear whether or not the investigators were measuring the accurate recall of information or of the rote repetition of information just immediately given. The distribution of counselee performance scores shows that 45% of counselees answered at least 9 out of 10 questions correctly and 78% of counselees answered at least 7 out of 10 questions correctly. This suggests that individual questions were not constructed so as to distinguish between individuals who were learning and those who were not. The distribution of counselee scores is markedly skewed, leading to a serious restriction of the variance of the scores and thus to a reduction of the reliability and, hence, the validity of the test. If individual questions are so easy that nearly everyone can answer them, then differences between individuals are probably due to error variance. This may lead to difficulties in analyzing and interpreting the data and conclusions based on such analyses need to be drawn cautiously.

At the beginning of the session, 35% of the counselees (n = 175) expressed feelings that were scored as negative, whereas at the end of the session 17% of counselees expressed such feelings. It is unclear whether or not this change is the result of the lowered anxiety that often occurs toward the end of a counseling session (or professional encounter in which bad news is not given) or was the result of the information provided in the session.

Rowley et al. (1984) and Lipkin et al. (1986) compared three different styles of genetic counseling—counseling provided by a trained physician (conventional counseling), videotaped counseling followed by an opportunity to question a trained physician (programmed counseling), and patient-structured counseling in which the content and affective tone of the counseling was said to be modulated according to the verbal and nonverbal responses of the counselee. The extent to which it was possible to "modulate" was constrained by the fact that the length of the session was restricted to 55 minutes and by the necessity to provide the same kind of information so as to match the length and content of the sessions provided by the other methods. In all three conditions, the counselors were male. The counselors in the patient-structured condition were internists with at least 1 year postresidency training in psychological medicine were said to provide psychologically sophisticated counseling.

The counselees consisted of asymptomatic individuals who were beta-thalassemia carriers detected in the course of screening. Subjects who participated in the research were randomly assigned to one of the three counseling methods so that each group was balanced as to age, sex, and marital and parental status. For each group, control persons who were negative for beta-thalassemia trait were matched to the experimental subjects, again, on the basis of age, sex, and marital and parental status.

Instead of counseling, control subjects were shown a film about taking care of their health that was about 55 minutes long. All subjects were tested before counseling (or before seeing the film) by questionnaires in which their knowledge of thalassemia and of genetics was assessed and in which information about medical experiences, attitudes about health, risk-taking attitudes, sexual satisfaction, marital satisfaction (Locke-Wallace test), and self-concept (Tennessee Self-Concept Test) were obtained. In addition, the Nowlis Mood Adjective Check List was administered. Immediately after the counseling or the film, subjects were retested for mood and their knowledge of thalassemia and genetics. Also, they were given the California Personality Inventory to take home and complete. At 2 months, subjects were retested for knowledge of thalassemia and of genetics, attitudes to risk taking, medical experience and attitudes, marital adjustment, and symptoms. The Shipley-Hartford test was also administered and a semistructured interview was conducted to assess additional reactions and actions not tapped by the questionnaires. At 10 months, the questionnaires were administered again and, instead of the Shipley-Hartford test, the Tennessee Self-Concept Test was given. At the end of the study, which ranged from 18 months for some subjects to 4 years for others, a semi-structured interview was conducted, and further questionnaires were administered to ascertain what the subjects "actually did as a result of counseling." The variable of interest was whether or not the subject at risk for thalassemia trait had shown "a rational response" by influencing others to be screened.

Although there were significant differences between experimental and control subjects on multiple measures (see the section on Rowley et al. (1984)), no significant differences were found between the different counseling approaches. The reasons for this are not readily apparent. Two hypotheses suggest themselves. First, the measures used (e.g., acquisition of information, mood) may not have been sensitive enough to differentiate between different styles of counseling. Second, the types of counseling may not have been as different as one might have supposed they were. The videotaped counseling was contaminated by the fact that a live person appeared at the end of the videotape and answered questions, and the psychologically sophisticated method might not have been so sophisticated. The counselors may not have had sufficient experience to provide "sophisticated" counseling. Also, each counseling method was constrained by time limitations and the need to present the same factual material. Thus, the fact that the counselors in the patient-structured approach asked about feelings may not have provided counselees with sufficient contrast to other methods since even in these sessions the major focus was on the factual, rather than the affective, content.

Comments

In their review, Evers-Kiebooms and van den Berghe (1979) suggested that researchers needed to conduct prospective studies and include control groups of uncounseled individuals to demonstrate the impact of genetic counseling. In the recent literature three prospective studies (Seidenfeld and Antley, 1981; Sorenson et al., 1981; Rowley et al., 1984) were reported and all demonstrated significant acquisition of risk information as a function of genetic counseling; the gains from before to after counseling ranged from 42% to nearly 300%. The largest study (Sorenson et al., 1981), in terms of its scope and the number of subjects studied, also demonstrated significant gains in the acquisition and recall of diagnostic information. The other studies employed a variety of different control groups. Black (1979) used a comparison group with a different, yet sufficiently similar, disorder as the experimental group (with a genetic disorder). However, the two groups were not comparable in their respective recurrence risks and other variables. Thus, when between-group differences occurred in recalling risk information, it was difficult to explain why. Her suggestion that the poorer recall of risk information among the parents of Down syndrome children may have been the consequence of lower salience of such information because of the availability of prenatal diagnosis seems counterintuitive. If anything, the availability of prenatal diagnosis might have made the risk information even more salient, at least for those counselees who would avail themselves of this technology (see the section on Ekwo et al. (1985), above). Oetting and Steele (1982) and Swerts (1987) used matched uncounseled control groups. In the latter study, significant differences were found between experimental and control persons in the recall of risk information, whereas in the former study no differences were found; an inadequately designed questionnaire may have contributed to the outcome in this study. Although in the study conducted by Ekwo et al. (1985), both experimental and control subjects received genetic counseling, the former group assented to and the other group declined amniocentesis. Thus, these investigators were able to study the educational effectiveness of counseling as a function of motivation to use or not use prenatal diagnosis.

In sum, the studies leave little or no doubt about the effectiveness of genetic counseling in educating counselees about diagnostic issues and recurrence risks. However, almost all the investigators suggest that there is room for improvement. In all the studies reviewed a substantial number of counselees either did not acquire or did not recall accurately the recurrence risk they received in counseling. In some cases this might have been due to the educational and other inadequacies counselees bring to the counseling session as well as insufficient motivation to acquire the information the counselor wishes to impart. Psychological defensiveness may also play a role in impeding the accurate acquisition and recall of factual information. The possibility also exists that there are deficiencies on the provider's end of things. The educational methods used by counselors may be inadequate to the task even when audio and visual aids are used. Counselors may not always be as clear in their explanations and presentation of information as they would like to believe they are. Also, considerable other information besides recurrence risks are provided to counselees during the course of genetic counseling that may, unwittingly, interfere with the acquisition of risk information.

In evaluating the success of the educational enterprise of genetic counseling, there has been an inordinate amount of attention given to the variables of risk and diagnosis. Thus, the learning of other important information (as for example, sources of medical and social support, infant stimulation programs, prognostic information) has not been adequately assessed. Recurrence risks may have less salience for some counselees than they have for genetic counselors. Such studies as that of Zorzi et al. (1980) suggest that the agendas and priorities of counselors and counselees may not always be concordant. The extent to which agenda discrepancies may contribute to communicational problems in counseling and, in turn, to later difficulties in factual recall needs further study.

It is unknown how much further room exists for improving the educational activities of genetic counselors without turning to other methods or means of providing counseling. In the one study (Rowley et al., 1984) in which different counseling modalities were compared, no significant differences emerged in educational effectiveness. This is an area of research that needs to be explored more thoroughly. It is possible that a ceiling may exist in improving the educational side of genetic counseling, and we possibly have already attained that ceiling. On the other hand, careful study of differing modalities, or combinations of modalities, modulating differing amounts of information, lengths of sessions, fitting particular counselors to specific counselees, etc., may prove to be more effective than current methods.

The role of cognitive processes in distorting acquired information and in using information for decision making needs to be better understood. Is precise recall of factual details and accurate probabilities really necessary for decision making? Perhaps a good-enough recall is all that may be needed for most persons. And good enough may be expressed in qualitative terms rather than quantitative ones. Lippman-Hand and Fraser (1979) have shown that counselees transform probabilities into qualitative form.

REPRODUCTION

Evers-Kiebooms and van den Berghe (1979) posed three questions regarding the impact of genetic counseling on reproduction: (1) Do counselees think that genetic counseling influenced their family planning? (2) What decisions do counselees make concerning reproduction after genetic counseling? (3) How many children were born after counseling in the different risk groups and what proportion was affected in the same way as the propositus? Since the last question is more in the provenance of the genetic epidemiologist than of the psychologist, no attempt will be made to deal with this question in the current review. However, the first two questions are of interest.

Asking counselees whether or not genetic counseling has influenced their family (or any other kind of) planning is fraught with pitfalls. How is the investigator, generally associated with the same group that provided the counseling and perhaps even the same individual, able to differentiate between the influence of counseling and the need of many counselees to please the provider and to make socially desirable responses? None of the studies conducted before or after 1979 have adequate controls for such responses. Thus, all reports of purported influence need to be viewed with some degree of caution. Furthermore, it is unclear what counselees mean when they say they have or have not been influenced by counseling. Counselees who reported being influenced have not necessarily reported that counseling assisted their formulation of reproductive plans or that their precounseling plans were changed as a consequence of counseling. In addition, counselees may not always be aware of being influenced by counseling even though they were. (Posthypnotic suggestions operate on this principle). Thus, there is a need to use outcome measures that do not depend on subjective awareness of influence, as for example, to conduct prospective studies so that measures of reproductive intentions or behavior prior to and at adequate periods after genetic counseling are obtained. It might then be possible to determine what proportion of counselees maintain or change their plans as a consequence of counseling. Even so, there are difficulties in discriminating between the effects of counseling and other sources of influence on an individual's or couple's reproductive plans and behavior.

Outcome Studies

Black (1979) studied 27 parents with a Down syndrome (DS) child and 20 parents with a child with mental retardation of unknown cause (UK) (see above). On post-counseling interviews, 11% of the former and 70% of the latter parents gave recurrence risks as a reason against further reproduction. Among the DS parents, 31% felt that the risk was an important consideration in decision making whereas among the UK parents 65% of the parents held this belief; 70% of the latter parents and 43% of the former ones sought genetic counseling because of concerns about recurrence risks.

Black also found that 50% of the 16 DS families and 40% of the 10 UK ones had a pregnancy since the birth of their affected children and that 20% of parents in each group (n = 25 for DS; n = 20 for UK) planned further children; 68% of the DS parents and 60% of the UK parents planned no further children. Because the recurrence risk for the UK parents (5%) as well as the severity of the retardation in their children was greater than that of the DS parents, it could not be said that the parents were responding only to their risks in their reproductive intentions and behavior. The reason most often given by the DS parents against additional children was that they had reached their desired family size; 52% of the 27 parents gave this reason. Among the 20 UK parents, 40% cited the burden of caring for a retarded child and 35% cited financial strains as the chief reasons against additional children. Only 35% of the UK parents cited reaching their desired family size as a reason against having more children; these parents were younger, on average, than the DS parents. The reasons for having additional children among both groups of parents included the desire for a large family (55% if the UK parents cited this reason) and other nongenetic motivations.

Lubs (1979) assessed family planning among individuals affected with either hemophilia or Duchenne muscular dystrophy, their spouses, and other relatives. Adults with at least a 5% risk of having an affected child and maternal aunts of the probands were included in the study; in all, 135 families were studied. By means of a post-counseling questionnaire it was found that 33% of the 76 males in the hemophilia families and 36% of the 22 males in the muscular dystrophy families had been sterilized because of the respective disease. Of the sterilized males in the hemophilia families, 13% (or 23% of all these males) were affected. Among the females, 9% in the hemophilia families (n = 186) and 7% in the muscular dystrophy families (n = 72) had been sterilized because of the disease. In 21% of couples, one or another spouse had been sterilized because of the disease. In addition, another 10% had been sterilized for reasons unrelated to the disease. The data are somewhat surprising since more than three-quarters of the males in the hemophilia families who had themselves sterilized were neither affected nor carriers of the disease whereas many of their spouses were at risk for being carriers.

In response to the question, "What is your feeling about limiting your family size because of the disease in your family?" 44% of the hemophilia family members and 40% of the muscular dystrophy ones responded, "No, the disease has not influenced the number of children I have or am planning to have"; 40% of the former and 50% of the latter family members responded, "Yes, because of the disease I have decided to limit my family size or adopt"; 16% of the hemophilia family members and 10% of the muscular dystrophy family members were undecided (n = 147 for hemophilia and n = 52 for muscular dystrophy).

Abramovsky et al. (1980) conducted a retrospective questionnaire study of families who had received genetic counseling (see above). Counselees were asked what their reproductive intentions had been prior to and after counseling and whether or not the counseling they received had influenced their decisions. Of 212 respondents, 57% said that their reproductive plans had been influenced by genetic counseling, 34% were not influenced, and 9% were undecided. Of the group who said they were influenced, 10% had originally planned not to have children and now were planning to have children, 60% maintained their precounseling decision and planned to have more children, 22% planned no further children (presumably this decision had already been made prior to counseling), and 8% planned to adopt a child. Of the respondents who said that their plans had not been influenced by genetic counseling, 57% planned more children, 4% changed their precounseling plans and now planned to have more children, 35% planned no more children, and 4% planned to adopt a child. Thus, irrespective of whether or not they thought they were influenced by counseling, counselees' reproductive plans remained relatively unchanged.

These investigators found an association between the magnitude of the recurrence risk and reproductive plans. Half of the 46 respondents who, according to the investigators, had a high risk and 37% of 22 respondents with a moderate risk planned to avoid pregnancy. However, 52% of 31 respondents who were not given a numeric risk (because no specific diagnosis was made) also planned to avoid pregnancy, suggesting that it was the subjective perception of risk rather than the objective risks which may have determined the outcome in this study.

Sorenson et al. (1981) studied the reproductive intentions of women before and following genetic counseling. About 61% of the women had a child with a birth defect or genetic abnormality; of these about 70% had a living child with a defect at the time of the study (see above for methods). Before counseling roughly one-third of the counselees stated that they planned a future pregnancy, one-third had no such plans, and one-third were not sure about their plans for further children. Little change was detected in stated reproductive intentions immediately after genetic counseling and 6 months later. At the latter time period, of 528 women studied, 44% reported that genetic counseling influenced their reproductive plans whereas 56% reported no such influence. Of the counselees who reported that genetic counseling influenced their reproductive plans, there was a 22% increase in the number of individuals who stated that they planned further pregnancies and a corresponding decrease in the number of women who were either unsure or who did not plan further pregnancies.

Sissine et al. (1981) conducted a retrospective questionnaire study of 200 families who received genetic counseling during a 4-year period. Collection of data occurred from 2 to 3 years after counseling for 75% and from 4 to 6 years later for 25% of the sample. Half of the group was also interviewed in their homes. Approximately 82% of the women and 75% of the men were under age 35 years at the time of the counseling; 51% of the group were Protestant and 44% were Roman Catholic. The outcome variables under study were reproductive attitudes, which included, among other things, reproductive intentions and behavior after counseling and feelings toward genetic counseling (positive, negative, or neutral). (Details as to how the responses about feelings and perceptions were converted into these latter categories were not given.) A sophisticated statistical analysis was made of the relationship of variables to pregnancy following counseling and four factors emerged as being significantly associated with pregnancy after counseling: pregnancy at the time of counseling, reproductive experience (e.g., having an affected child, living or deceased), the woman's age, and the given level of risk. Almost all couples who were pregnant when they were counseled initiated another pregnancy after counseling. Couples who had a miscarriage, stillbirth, or whose affected child died were more likely to begin a postcounseling pregnancy than couples with other reproductive histories. Also, couples with relatively fewer children were more likely to initiate a pregnancy after counseling than couples with two or more children. These findings suggest that the parental desire for children is a major determinant of postcounseling reproductive behavior. It was also found that couples with high genetic risks were less likely to initiate a postcounseling pregnancy than those with low risks. (High and low risks were not defined by the investigators.) However, further analysis supported the view that the parental desire for children and past reproductive history, rather than recurrence risks, accounted for the data.

Oetting and Steele (1982) carried out a questionnaire and interview study of 23 matched pairs of families with a Down syndrome child; half the families had received genetic counseling following the birth of the child and half had not (see above for methods). These investigators found no significant differences in reproduction between counseled and noncounseled families. Among the counseled families, 17 (74%) stated that genetic counseling had no effect on their subsequent reproductive decisions.

Wertz et al. (1984) studied the reproductive plans of 836 women before and immediately after genetic counseling (see Sorenson et al. (1981), above, for details on methods). Prior to counseling about one-third of the counselees were unsure about their reproductive plans over the next 2 years. Following counseling there was a 22% decrease of uncertainty in this group, suggesting that genetic counseling was effective in reducing the uncertainty among persons who, on self-report, were uncertain about further reproduction. However, this gain was offset somewhat by the fact that among the 555 counselees who were certain about their reproductive plans before counseling, 63 had become unsure of their plans after counseling. Thus, overall there was a net gain of certainty of about 6% as a result of genetic counseling. Of 646 fertile counselees who remained in the study 6 months later, about 34% were uncertain about their reproductive plans; certainty decreased (nonsignificantly) from 71% immediately after counseling to 66% at the 6 months follow-up. In other words, certainty and uncertainty remained stable over time.

Associated strongly with postcounseling uncertainty were the following variables: precounseling uncertainty and uncertainty about the ideal family size the person wanted to achieve; counselees who came to genetic counseling unsure of their reproductive plans or of their ideal family size generally left counseling still uncertain. Also, counselees who had stronger concerns about the effects of an affected child on one's social life or had serious problems caring for an affected child at home were significantly more likely to be uncertain about their reproductive plans after counseling than counselees who did not have such concerns or difficulties. Wertz et al. (1984) concluded that genetic counseling was not effective in facilitating reproductive decision making. Furthermore, they argued that genetic counseling may not be a viable means of reducing reproductive uncertainty for many counselees. However, they point out that 78% of the counselees with uncertain reproductive plans prior to counseling had indicated that they came for counseling to obtain information for making a reproductive decision. Of these, 65% remained uncertain about their plans after counseling; 6 months later, however, this dropped to 48% of those remaining in the study. This suggests that the effects of genetic counseling on the issues underlying uncertainty may not be felt immediately after counseling. Rather, it may be part of an ongoing process, over time, of evaluation, weighing of options, and of responses to personal and interpersonal factors all of which contribute to reproductive decision making.

How does certainty and uncertainty about reproductive plans translate into actual behavior? Wertz and Sorenson (1983) studied contraceptive use among 648 fertile counselees 6 months after genetic counseling. Among the counselees who were reproductively uncertain 94% were using contraceptives, which, on inspection, was similar to the contraceptive use among counselees who intended to have no children (92%) as well as those who wanted a child but not within the next 2 years (89%). Among counselees who intended to have a child within 2 years of the counseling, 63% were using contraceptives.

Counselees who stated immediately after genetic counseling that they were unsure about their reproductive plans may have had more ambivalence about having further children than counselees who were reproductively certain. Thus, it might be expected that the former might have a higher contraceptive failure rate than the latter. Indeed, the uncertain counselees showed less effective contraceptive use than the counselees who were certain did. The contraceptive failure rate among counselees who were certain they wanted to prevent a pregnancy was 2%; and among those who intended to have a child, but not within the next 2 years, it was 4%; among the reproductively uncertain group it was 10%. It is not clear whether or not these contraceptive "failures" might have been the result of changes in reproductive intentions.

Rowley et al. (1984) (see above for methods) studied 142 individuals who had been detected as being beta-thalassemia trait carriers. Before genetic counseling, each subject completed the Locke-Wallace Marital Adjustment Scale and other questionnaires. Compared to a matched group of control subjects negative for beta-thalassemia trait, the experimental subjects showed a significantly better marital adjustment and, on self-report, greater sexual activity and satisfaction than control persons 10 months after counseling. The latter showed a 7% decrease in sexual activity whereas the experimentals showed a 12% increase ($P < .01$).

From 18 months to 4 years after they had received genetic counseling, subjects were interviewed and completed a further questionnaire (Lipkin et al., 1986). All but one of the subjects were found to have informed at least one other person about the counseling and their trait status and 43% were said to have "caused" 106 other persons to be screened for beta-thalassemia trait. Of the latter, 32% were spouses, 22% were sibs, and 34% were children; the remainder were other relatives and in-laws. Subjects were likely to have someone else screened if they were fertile and planning to have children. As one might expect, younger subjects were more likely than older ones to have had someone screened. Also, subjects who had a high score on a test of thalassemia knowledge immediately after counseling and who had relatively higher levels of education were more likely to have another person screened than individuals with low scores and lesser education.

The investigators apparently were disappointed in the level of preventive intervention following genetic counseling, since 57% of subjects did not have anyone else screened. Because there was no comparable group of uncounseled subjects, there was no way of knowing how successful or unsuccessful the counseling had been.

Sorenson et al. (1987) studied the reproductive plans of 185 fecund women who were at risk for children with birth defects and genetic disorders not amenable to prenatal diagnosis (see above). Before genetic counseling about 40% of the women said that they intended a pregnancy. Broken down by risk level, 52% of 92 counselees with a risk of 10% or less, and 27% of 93 counselees with a risk of over 10% said they intended a pregnancy. Six months after counseling, 60% of the former group and 42% of the latter group said that they intended a pregnancy (this includes women who became pregnant in the period following counseling). Overall about 52% of the women were intending a pregnancy 6 months after counseling. Proportionately there was a 15% increase among the women with the relatively lower risks and a 56% increase among the counselees with a relatively higher risk. The major variable associated with postcounseling reproductive intentions was the counselee's precounseling reproductive plans. The level of risk was not found to be strongly associated with changes in reproductive intentions from before counseling to 6 months after counseling.

Swerts (1987) (see above) studied 51 couples in which the woman was not pregnant at the time of genetic counseling. All couples had had a child with a neural tube defect. After counseling, 70% of the couples said, on interview, that they were undecided about having more children and were now thinking of doing so; 10% had decided to have no further children before counseling and also decided, after counseling, to have more children. Of the couples who were undecided about children before counseling, only 2% decided to have no more children after counseling; 8% were still undecided about reproduction; 10% of the couples stated that their pre-counseling decision had not changed. Thus, at least 80% of the couples said that the information received in genetic counseling influenced them to decide to have more children. Swerts reported that 86% of the couples reached a decision about children almost immediately after the genetic counseling and that for 56% of couples (n = 41) the most influential topic discussed during the counseling on their decision was the availability of prenatal diagnosis. Miller et al. (1987) studied the reproductive patterns of men affected with hemophilia and carrier women; these subjects may have had more than one counseling session over a 6-year study period, although 7% of the former may not have received counseling at all. During counseling, the affected men were presented with several options: having no children, having children, prenatal sex detection with abortion of carrier females, and artificial insemination (AID). Carrier females were presented with the options of not having children, of taking the risk, considering adoption, and prenatal sex detection with abortion of affected males. The investigators pointed out that attempts were made to keep the counseling nondirective and to give each reproductive option equal weight.

It was found that two-thirds of 132 affected males 25 years of age and older had married and of these 62% had children. Only 3% of the married men with hemophilia chose to adopt a child, 1% chose AID, and none chose the option of aborting a carrier female. Among the 39 carrier females studied there were 49 pregnancies, 65% of which had occurred after the initial counseling. Prenatal diagnosis was chosen in about half of the pregnancies, and the investigators seemed to feel that this response rate might have been due to the "more thorough counseling" they provided.

Shiloh and Saxe (1989) studied, by questionnaire, a group of 33 couples and 10 individuals before and after genetic counseling and measured reproductive intentions on a seven-point scale in response to the question, "Do you intend to have a child (or another child if now pregnant) at any time in the future?" Responses ranged from "definitely yes" to "definitely no." These workers found that of 73 counselees, 48% did not change their precounseling reproductive intentions, 37% said that they intended more children, and 15% said that they intended to have less children. Overall, for those who changed their intentions after counseling, there was a small but significant increase in the number of counselees intending further children.

Process Studies

Wertz and Sorenson (1986) found that almost 44% of women reported that their reproductive plans for the next 2 years had been influenced by the genetic counseling they had received 6 months previously (see sections on Sorenson et al. (1981)). Of these, 53% maintained their original reproductive plans, 15% intended more preg-nancies, and 13% intended fewer pregnancies than they intended prior to counseling. About 19% of the counselees were uncertain about their plans for children. Analysis of the data showed that the women who said that they were influenced by the coun-seling session came to counseling to obtain information about whether or not to have a child, had discussed this decision in depth with the genetic counselor, and tended to be better educated than women who said they were not influenced by the counseling. The pattern of change or stability of reproductive plans among the women who said they were not influenced by the genetic counseling was the same as that among those who were influenced. These findings suggest that many counselees may use genetic counseling as a way of legitimizing or receiving professional sanction for a decision already taken prior to counseling. The impact or influence of genetic counseling on reproductive decisions, at least the counseling studied by Wertz and Sorenson (1986), was not substantial.

Sorenson and Wertz (1986) studied the agreement between spouses about repro-ductive plans before and after genetic counseling. On a self-administered question-naire, each counselee was asked to indicate their reproductive plans within the next 2 years and also longer term; data were analyzed on couples where neither partner was sterilized and the wife was still in her childbearing years. Before counseling, 74% of 542 couples agreed about their reproductive plans for the next 2 years and 63% agreed about their longer-term plans. About 7–10 days after genetic counseling the couple was asked to fill out the questionnaire again, and it was found that there were no significant changes in agreement either about short- or long-term reproduc-tive plans. These data suggest that for the approximately 25% of couples who had dis-agreements about reproductive plans prior to counseling, these disagreements were not resolved by the counseling.

Furthermore, couples disagreeing about reproduction were also likely to disagree about other important issues pertaining to perceptions about genetic disorders and ge-netic counseling. It is conceivable that the postcounseling measures were taken too soon after the counseling and more time might have been needed for a consensus to be reached.

Shiloh and Saxe (1989) (see above) found that postcounseling reproductive inten-tions was more highly correlated with subjective perceptions of risk ($r = -0.41$) than with objective risks ($r = -0.07$). The higher the perceived risk, the lower the repro-ductive intention; the finding held for both male and female counselees.

Comments

What impact does genetic counseling have on the reproductive decisions and behav-ior of counselees? One approach to this question is to determine whether or not coun-selees believe that counseling has influenced them. The data dealing with this area span a wide range. In one study (Oetting and Steele, 1982), only 26% of counselees believed that counseling had affected their reproductive decisions, whereas, in an-other (Abramovsky et al., 1980), 57% believed that they had been influenced. In both these studies, subjects were required to recall feelings and thoughts in the relatively distant past, and, in both, changes in reproductive intentions were not related to being influenced by counseling. Sorenson et al. (1981) found that 44% of counselees thought that their reproductive plans has been influenced by counseling that had occurred only 6 months earlier. In this instance, there was an increase in the number of planned pregnancies. Overall, in this reviewer's opinion, the findings of these studies provide little or no insight into how genetic counseling had made a difference, if at all, in the decision making of counselees.

A different approach to the initial question is to determine what the reproductive intentions of counselees were before counseling and again after counseling. Changes in plans, other things being equal, might possibly be attributed to the counseling. Studied prospectively, it becomes apparent that a vast number of counselees already have formulated reproductive plans prior to counseling and, in general, counseling does not seem to alter such plans in a major way. The results of several studies (Sissine et al., 1981; Wertz et al., 1984; Sorenson et al., 1987; Swerts, 1987) indicate that precounseling reproductive intentions play a major, if not *the* major, role in determining postcounseling reproductive plans, This suggests that for many counselees, the role of counseling largely is to confirm or reinforce a decision already taken rather than to shape a reproductive decision from the onset.

If precounseling intentions are such a major determinant of later reproductive decisions, what role do recurrence risks play in these decisions? The answer is hardly straightforward. In some studies (Black, 1979; Abramovsky et al., 1980), counselees stated that recurrence risks were a major consideration in their decisions about children. Also, older studies, summarized by Evers-Kiebooms and van den Berghe (1979), suggest that relatively higher risks tend to deter reproduction more so than do lower risks. However, counselees' perceptions of a given genetic disorder are often complex. To tease out the influence of risk from other factors (under the general heading of burden) may be difficult, if not impossible (Leonard et al., 1972; Lippman-Hand and Fraser, 1979). The overall gestalt of a disorder may have a more profound impact on the thinking of counselees than any one piece (such as risk) in isolation. Future research may need to adopt different strategies (e.g., in-depth interviews of counselees before, during, and after decision making) than those used heretofore to clarify this matter.

An important study on the relationship between recurrence risks and reproductive intentions is that of Sorenson et al. (1987) (see above), who focused on counselees at risk for disorders in which prenatal diagnosis was not available, minimizing or removing this variable from the decision-making "equation." Separated by risk levels, these investigators found that the postcounseling reproductive intentions of counselees with high risks showed relatively greater change over time than those of counselees with low risks. The change was in the direction of more, not less, children. These data cast some doubt on the negative influence of recurrence risks on reproductive decisions. Obviously, the relationship between recurrence risks and reproduction decisions requires further elucidation. Future research needs to determine how counselees process risk information and use it, if at all, in their decision-making processes.

In some circles, the view has been expressed that genetic counseling subserved negative eugenics goals. The data reviewed here suggests that this view may be incorrect. Several studies (Abramovsky et al., 1980; Sorenson et al., 1981, 1987; Shiloh and Saxe, 1989) indicate that there is a net increase, not decrease in the desire for children following genetic counseling.

Could it be that one of the functions of counseling is to reduce the reproductive anxieties of counselees? In other counseling contexts it is known that when counselees discuss anxiety and fear-ridden subjects, they tend to feel relief afterwards, even if their objective behavior seems to remain unchanged. A similar phenomenon, the so-called risky shift effect, has been described by social psychologists (Rettig, 1966; Chandler and Rabow, 1969; Pearn, 1979). Does the discussion of their chances of having an affected child, in itself, serve to reduce the reproductive anxiety of counselees at risk for genetic disorders, independent of whatever information is conveyed to them? Does this reduction then lead to an increased desire for children?

The findings of Rowley et al. (1984) regarding the increase of sexual activity following genetic counseling also deserve confirmation since the finding is consistent with the apparent increase in desire for more children after counseling.

The studies also suggest an intriguing possibility regarding the relationship between risk perceptions and reproductive intentions. It has always been assumed that causality in this instance flows from risk perception to reproductive intention, that is, risks influence decisions.

However, the causal flow may be in the opposite direction, that is, risk perceptions may be ex post facto justifications of decisions already taken or a rationale of one's perceived behavior (Slovic, 1987). This topic will be taken up again in a subsequent publication dealing with risk perception.

ACKNOWLEDGMENTS

The reviewer wishes to thank Dr. Arthur Falek for his helpful suggestions.

REFERENCES

Abramovsky I, Godmilow L, Hirschhorn K, Smith H (1980) Analysis of a follow-up study of genetic counseling. Clin Genet 17:1–12.

Black RB (1979) The effects of diagnostic uncertainty and available options on perceptions of risk. Birth Defects: Original Article Series 15(5C):341–354.

Chandler S, Rabow J (1969) Ethnicity and acquaintance as variables in risk-taking. J Soc Psychol 77:221–229.

Childs B (1978) Genetic counseling: a critical review of the published literature. In: Cohen BH, Lilienfeld AM, Huang PC (eds). Genetic Issues in Public Health and Medicine. Springfield, IL: CC Thomas, pp 329–357.

Ekwo EE, Seals BF, Kim JO, Williamson RA, Hanson JW (1985) Factors influencing maternal estimates of genetic risk. Am J Med Genet 20:491–504.

Evers-Kiebooms G, van den Berghe H (1979) The impact of genetic counseling: a review of published follow-up studies. Clin Genet 15:465–474.

Evers-Kiebooms G, Vlietinck R, Fryns JP, van den Berghe H (1984) Impact on family planning of the birth of a child with 21 trisomy. In: Berg MJ (ed). Perspectives and Progress in Mental Retardation, Vol. 2. Baltimore: University Park Press, pp 323–333.

Hsia YE (1977) Approaches to the appraisal of genetic counseling. In: Lubs H, de la Cruz F (eds). Genetic Counseling. New York: Raven Press, pp 53–81.

Keltikangas-Jarvinen L, Autio S (1983) Psychological obstacles to genetic education. Scand J Soc Med 11:7–10.

Leonard CO, Chase G, Childs B (1972) Genetic counseling: a consumer's view. N Engl J Med 287:433–439.

Lipkin M, Fisher L, Rowley PT, Loader S, Iker HP (1986) Genetic counseling of asymptomatic carriers in a primary care setting. Ann Intern Med 105:115–123.

Lippman-Hand A, Fraser FC (1979) Genetic counseling: parents' responses to uncertainty. In: Epstein CJ, Curry CJR, Packman S, Sherman S, Hall BD (eds). Risk, Communication, and Decision Making in Genetic Counseling. Birth Defects: Original Article Series 15(5C): 325–340.

Lubs ML (1979) Does genetic counseling influence risk attitudes and decision making? In: Epstein CJ, Curry CJR, Packman S, Sherman S, Hall BD (eds). Risk, Communication, and Decision Making in Genetic Counseling. Birth Defects: Original Article Series 15(5C): 355–367.

Miller CH, Hilgartner MW, Aledort LM (1987) Reproductive choices in hemophilic men and carriers. Am J Med Genet 26:591–598.

Oetting LA, Steele NM (1982) A controlled retrospective follow-up study of the impact of genetic counseling on parental reproduction following the birth of a Down syndrome child. Clin Genet 21:7–13.

Pearn J (1979) Decision making and reproductive choice. In: Hsia YE, Hirschhorn K, Silverberg RL, Godmilow L (eds). Counseling in Genetics. New York: Alan R. Liss, Inc., pp 223–238.

Rettig S (1966) Group discussion and predicted ethical risk taking. J Pers Soc Psychol 3:629–633.

Rowley PT, Lipkin M, Fisher L (1984) Screening and genetic counseling for beta-thalassemia trait in a population unselected for interest: comparison of three counseling methods. Am J Hum Genet 36:677–689.

Seidenfeld MJ, Antley RM (1981) Genetic counseling: a comparison of counselee's genetic knowledge before and after (Part III). Am J Med Genet 10:107–112.

Shaw M (1977) Review of published studies of genetic counseling: a critique of methodology. In: Lubs H, de la Cruz F (eds). Genetic Counseling. New York: Raven Press, pp 35–49.

Shiloh S, Saxe L (1989) Perception of recurrence risk by genetic counselees. Psychol Health 3:45–61.

Sissine FJ, Rosser L, Steele MW, Marchese S, Garver KL, Berman N (1981) Statistical analysis of genetic counseling impacts. Eval Rev 5:745–757.

Slovic P (1987) Perception of risk. Science 236:280–285.

Sorenson JR, Wertz DC (1986) Couple agreement before and after genetic counseling. Am J Med Genet 25:549–555.

Sorenson JR, Swazey JP, Scotch NA (1981) Reproductive Pasts, Reproductive Futures: Genetic Counseling and Its Effectiveness. Birth Defects: Original Article Series 17(4):1–192.

Sorenson JR, Scotch NA, Swazey JP, Wertz DC, Heeren TC (1987) Reproductive plans of genetic counseling clients not eligible for prenatal diagnosis. Am J Med Genet 28:345–352.

Swerts A (1987) Impact of genetic counseling and prenatal diagnosis for Down Syndrome and neural tube defects. Birth Defects: Original Article Series 23(2):61–83.

Wertz DC, Sorenson JR (1983) Contraceptive use and efficacy in a genetically counseled population. Soc Biol 30:328–334.

Wertz DC, Sorenson JR (1986) Client reactions to genetic counseling: self-reports of influence. Clin Genet 30:494–502.

Wertz DC, Sorenson JR, Heeren TC (1984) Genetic counseling and reproductive uncertainty. Am J Med Genet 18:79–88.

Whitten CF, Thomas JF, Nishiura EN (1981) Sickle cell trait counseling—evaluation of counselors and counselees. Am J Hum Genet 33:802–816.

Zorzi G, Thurman SK, Kistenmacher ML (1980) Importance and adequacy of genetic counseling information: impressions of parents with Down's syndrome children. Ment Retard 18:255–257.

10

Teaching and Counseling[1]

There are two basic approaches to genetic counseling, education (here called the teaching model) and counseling. Genetic counselors often attempt to combine aspects of both approaches with, I suggest, limited success, since the fundamental philosophies and professional demands of each approach seldom mesh and their differences tend to exceed their commonalities. In this paper, I will review my understanding of these two approaches and underscore the need for acquiring specific skills in order to deal with the unique issues that arise in genetic counseling.

THE TEACHING MODEL

Table 10.1 shows the goal and underlying assumptions of the teaching model of genetic counseling. The model is based on the perception that clients come to genetic counseling primarily to obtain information (Hsia, 1979).The role of the professional is to provide information and correct misinformation and misperceptions. The specific information to be conveyed is often determined by the issues and questions the counselee raises and, unless there are institutional constraints, is often left up to the professional's judgment.

The teaching model tends to assume that human beings act and make decisions in a more or less rational manner and, when informed, clients should be able to make their own decisions.

The assumptions made about human behavior and psychology in the model tend to be simplified and minimized. For example, personality variables are not generally taken into account in professional–client interactions and past psychological history of

[1]This essay first appeared Kessler S (1997) Psychological aspects of genetic counseling. IX. Teaching and counseling. *Journal of Genetic Counseling* 6:287–295. Reprinted with kind permission of the publisher, Kluwer Academic/Human Sciences Press.

Table 10.1. The Teaching Model

1. Goal: educated counselees.
2. Based on perception that clients come for information.
3. The model assumes that if informed, clients should be able to make their own decisions.
4. Assumptions about human behavior and psychology simplified and minimized; cognitive and rational processes are emphasized.
5. Counseling task is to provide information as impartially and a balanced as possible; correct misinformation.
6. Education is an end in itself.
7. Relationship with client based on authority rather than mutuality.

the client is not given great weight. It probably does not change the kind of information one provides if the client had been raped a year earlier or if a parent died several weeks before the consultation.

If the style of teaching is basically a professional monologue (what might be called the lecture-hall type), as it often is, individual differences do not play a great role. Thus, the professional has the tendency to provide more or less the same information to all counselees—one size fits all (Brunger and Lippman, 1995)—a decided advantage where there is a high volume of patients. This tendency is ironic given how important individual differences are in understanding genetic variation. Nonetheless, it has an apparent efficiency that makes it attractive in a busy clinic.

The relationship between the teacher and student is by definition an unequal one (Kenen and Smith, 1995); the teacher is the more knowing one and the student is the learner. This has psychological consequences. It creates interactions in which personal engagement with clients is minimized and little room is left for the expression of their autonomy and individuality. Autonomy may actually be suppressed. This, in turn, tends to increase the dependency on the professional's authority and is likely to lead to requests for advice and opinion (Kessler, 1992).

Emotional responses under the teaching model tend to be seen as interferences with the learning process and so the professional tends to use emotionally suppressive techniques, as, for example, changing the subject when emotionality threatens to emerge or refraining from asking emotionally evocative questions. Whether or not such strategies are employed deliberately, they do tend to be effective. However, they set a tone that might interfere with a counseling approach should the professional attempt to change to that role later in the session.

Under the teaching model the professional tries to achieve neutrality, even-handedness, impartiality, and noncoerciveness, and these terms may be more appropriate as ideals and more descriptive of the procedures in the model than the more psychologically loaded term, nondirectiveness (Kessler, 1996).

THE COUNSELING MODEL

Table 10.2 shows the goals and assumptions of the counseling model. There are multiple interrelated goals to achieve in the model. Perhaps the most difficult one of all is to engage and understand the other person since all operational aspects of the model proceed from that understanding. The professional also attempts to bolster and reinforce the counselee's sense of competence and capacity for autonomy. This is accomplished in one or more of several ways, but mostly by deliberately providing space and time for counselees to feel they have progressively greater control over the agenda of the genetic counseling session. Not full control, mind you, but sufficient control so that counselees feel they are shaping the interaction. The professional's task is to create conditions within the session that encourage the counselees to be active in their own behalf. This is discussed further below.

The counseling model is based on the perception that counselees come for counseling for complex reasons—above and beyond the need for information—and the model makes complex assumptions about human behavior and psychology. For example, the counselor might assume that counselees strive for self-actualization or are conflict-driven as, for instance, when they attempt to achieve contradictory goals (e.g., protecting a fetus versus the need to give birth to a healthy child). Also, under this model, the counselor is active in eliciting any latent issues that the clients bring with them to counseling.

The counseling tasks in the model are multiple and require the counselor to assess the counselees' strengths and limitations, needs, values, and decisional trends. The model requires a range of counseling skills and an individualized counseling style to fit the counselee's needs and agendas.

Notice that the primary goal of the counseling model is not to educate the counselees and when education is necessary, as it generally is in genetic counseling, it is used as a means to achieve other (psychological) goals, not for its own sake. Education is not considered an end in itself.

Table 10.2. The Counseling Model

1. Goals
   a. To understand the other person
   b. To bolster their inner sense of competence
   c. To promote a greater sense of control over their lives
   d. Relieve psychological distress, if possible
   e. To support and possibly raise their self-esteem
   f. To help them find solutions to specific problems
2. Based on perception that clients come for counseling for complex reasons (e.g., information, validation, support, anxiety reduction).
3. The model has complex assumptions about human behavior and psychology that are brought to bear in counseling.
4. Counseling tasks complex
   a. Requires assessment of client's strengths and limitations, needs, values, and decision trends
   b. Requires range of counseling skills to achieve goals
   c. Requires individualized counseling style to fit client's needs and agendas; flexibility
   d. Requires counselor to attend to and take care of his or her own inner life
5. Education is used as a means to achieve above goals.
6. Relationship aims for mutuality.

THE MODELS COMPARED

Table 10.3 shows a possible difference between the teaching and counseling models in response to the question, "What do most people generally do in our situation?"

Both responses are educational, but what the professional says and how it is said differs considerably in the two approaches. The teaching response tends to be filled with facts and figures, something conspicuously absent in the counseling approach. This is not to say that the latter approach is any less deliberate or precise than the former. On the contrary, there may be as much precision in the choice of tone and words in the counseling approach as there is in the teaching model. However, the goals achieved and the impact on the counselees are different.

The teaching model emphasizes the authority of the professional, something that gets reinforced as each fresh detail is presented, whereas the counseling model response de-emphasizes this aspect of the relationship without the professional relinquishing any authority. Also, the teaching model tends to promote psychological passivity—a self-defeating strategy when the professional wants to encourage others to make their own decisions—as the professional keeps repeating the message, "See how much I know and how little you do." The net psychological impact of this strategy is to enrich the authority, status, and ego of the professional at the expense of the client. The purpose of any counseling strategy is to reverse this process and leave the client psychologically enriched even if it is at the expense of the professional. In contrast to the teaching model, the latter strategy tends to make room for the active expression of the autonomy, individuality, and self-directedness of the counselees.

Counseling professionals tend to ally themselves with the counselees' problem rather than distancing themselves as the teaching professional tends to do in the above example. This is experienced on the client's side as empathy, something noticeably absent or minimized in the teaching approach. The quality of the empathy offered is such as to encourage the counselees to be psychologically active since the underlying message is one of, "I'll be there with you in case you stumble."

Table 10.3. Comparison of Teaching and Counseling Approaches in Response to the Question, "What Do Most People Generally Do in Our Situation?"

Teaching Model
Well, something like 94.3% (fictitious figure) of the counselees we see in our clinic terminate pregnancies. However, remember, this figure only applies to our clinic and not to other clinics. Their figures may differ from ours by as much as 10%. Also, remember that the counselees we see may not represent an unbiased sampling of all couples in your situation and may be more likely to terminate a pregnancy than couples in the general population. Do you have any other questions?

Counseling Model
Most people in your situation face the same dilemmas and hard choices you are probably facing. Each couple wrestles with the same questions and some decide one way others to the other way according to their personal goals and needs. I wish these decisions were easier to make but they are not; each couple seems to have to go through their own struggle and find the solution that feels right and fits best for them. Any way I can help you make and live with that decision I'll sure help try.

DISCUSSION

The teaching model is an inheritance from the past when genetic counseling activities were mostly concentrated in academic departments and among a handful of academic physicians (Ludmerer, 1972). It is a powerful model and, to a point, it succeeds in its goals. Considerable data suggest that, in broad outline, many consumers assimilate the information they receive, especially around the issues of risk and diagnosis (Sorenson et al., 1981). The same data also indicate that the teaching approach leaves a considerable number of consumers uninformed or poorly informed, a finding that is not surprising given that, at least to my knowledge, professionals largely are not trained in pedagogical skills. Why training programs have not paid more attention to the teaching aspects of genetic counseling is puzzling given the centrality the teaching model seems to play in the work situation.

The teaching model has certain limitations. First, it tends to lead to excessive information giving, which might be appropriate in the classroom setting but is hardly so in the consultation room. In my experience, consumers frequently receive far too much information, more than most people can assimilate and understand. This too may be the result of inadequate training in the skills of teaching on the part of the professional, but it might also represent work-related pressures.

Second, when the professional shifts attention away from information to questions of personal meaning and to discussions of the consequences of the information they have conveyed that the inadequacies of the teaching model become apparent. The skills of pedagogy become largely irrelevant at that point. The counseling model is also a powerful model of professional–client interactions. However, given the structure of the field, especially in terms of who defines the specific work of (and hires and fires) genetic counselors, total reliance on a counseling model may not be feasible.

The strength of the counseling model resides in dealing with personal and interpersonal issues, the subjective meaning of information (e.g., situations in which the results of predictive testing are given), and such other psychological issues as decision making, nondirectiveness, etc. Its greatest limitation is that it requires a great deal from the professional. First of all, it requires an unusual set of skills. Counseling is not about listening to and "tut-tutting" about the other's adversities. It is basically about understanding the other person and providing appropriate help in the form of how to think about and work through life problems. This is accomplished in a way that empowers the person, fosters their autonomy, and evokes their competency. Among the skills that need to be acquired and honed are those in which one trains oneself to subordinate his or her personal angst, values, and beliefs and keep the other person and their inner world in the mental foreground. This requires hours of practice and discipline, not dissimilar to the process of learning to master a musical instrument.

Second, the counseling model requires the professional to inhibit and suppress one's own needs (for power, status, recognition, authority, etc.) for the sake of someone else. This means the development of attitudes and mature ways of thinking about one's professional role that promote the subordination of the professional's normal ego satisfactions and needs. Some parents learn such skills in the process of raising children, which generally calls for the selfless giving of oneself. In the counseling situation, these needs are intensified.

Last, the counseling model is limited in application by external circumstances. For example, changes in the health delivery system in which efficiency, profit, or other factors rather than the needs of clients dictate what transpires in professional–client interactions will clearly make the counseling model more difficult to use. But, even in such circumstances, creative professionals will find ways, as they always have, to retain the human side of their work. This might require the acquisition and development of rapid means of assessing others and understanding their needs, the skills seasoned professionals tend to develop in any case.

In this paper, I have tried to differentiate between the goals, philosophies, and procedures of teaching and counseling. A teacher needs to organize and present a mass of details in a comprehensive, clear, and understandable way to the other person. This requires planning as well as the knowledge of pedagogical skills. Counselors need to learn very different skills as, for example, how to retain one's mental focus on the other person rather than on one's own thoughts and feelings and how to make each thing said or done contribute to bolstering the client's self-esteem, competence, and autonomy. In counseling, the self is subordinated to the other's needs. The capacity for empathy is not a necessity for a teacher—although it would be nice to have it—whereas it is essential for a counselor.

The two models also have a differential impact on the professional. The counseling model requires that the counselor attends to and take care of his or her own inner life; this is in sharp contrast to the teaching model, which makes little psychological demand on the professional.

In the training of genetic counselors, insufficient attention has been given to how the two models described here might be learned and put to effective professional use. The skill demands of the teaching model tend to reinforce attitudes and procedures antithetical to those required in counseling. This may be confusing to students and interfere with their ability to learn and perfect either pedagogical or counseling skills. As working professionals, many may find themselves relying heavily on a teaching approach, further reinforcing behaviors that interfere with the development of the counseling skills needed to help clients reach decisions, deal with couple's conflicts, manage guilt and shame, provide empathy, and, in general, maintain a nondirective stance.

In sum, the skills needed for teaching and counseling differ so vastly, they require an unusually gifted and flexible professional to combine them both in the shortterm interactions of genetic counseling. But, this, in a nutshell, is the challenge of the profession.

ACKNOWLEDGMENTS

I would like to thank Ms. Liz Stierman for reading an earlier version of this paper and for her constructive suggestions.

REFERENCES

Brunger F, Lippman A (1995) Resistance and adherence to the norms of genetic counseling. J Genet Counsel 4:151–167.

Hsia YE (1979) The genetic counselor as information giver. In: Capron AM, Lappe M, Murray RF, Powledge TM, Twiss SB, Bergsma D (eds). Genetic Counseling: Facts, Values, and Norms. Birth Defects: Original Article Series 15(2):169–186, New York: Alan R. Liss.

Kenen RH, Smith ACM (1995) Genetic counseling for the next 25 years: models for the future. J Genet Counsel 4:115–124.

Kessler S (1989) Psychological aspects of genetic counseling. VI. A critical review of the literature dealing with education and reproduction. Am J Med Genet 34:340–353.

Kessler S (1992) Psychological aspects of genetic counseling. VII. Thoughts on directiveness. J Genet Counsel 1:9–17.

Kessler S (1996) Nondirectiveness Revisited. Talk given October 27, 1996 at 15th Annual Educational Conference of The National Society of Genetic Counselors, San Francisco, CA.

Ludmerer KM (1972) Genetics and American Society. Baltimore: Johns Hopkins University Press.

Sorenson JR, Swazey JP, Scotch NA (1981) Reproductive Pasts, Reproductive Futures: Genetic Counseling and Its Effectiveness. Birth Defects: Original Article Series 17(4):1–192. New York: Alan R. Liss.

11

Thoughts on Directiveness[1]

INTRODUCTION

The terms "directiveness" and "nondirectiveness" have been part of the lexicon of genetic counseling for many decades. Yet, one has little confidence that a consensus exists about the meanings given to these terms. Simply put, when counselor A says that he is being nondirective, is he doing and saying things comparable to counselor B, who says that she is being nondirective? In the virtual absence of empirical information on what transpires in genetic counseling sessions, the only honest answer we can give is that we do not know. Clearly, our operational understanding of directiveness and nondirectiveness is limited. Similar things also might be said about related terms, such as "prescriptive" counseling (Antley, 1979), and "guidance" (Pauker and Pauker, 1979; Czeizel et al., 1981), which to some seem more palatable proxies for directiveness.

In the early history of genetic counseling, directive counseling may have been the rule. Attempts to eschew the influence of the eugenics movement led to the development of nondirective approaches. By the end of the 1960s, nondirective genetic counseling had become firmly established, at least in the United States, and by the end of the 1980s, almost 90% of medical geneticists in 17 different countries endorsed nondirective positions (Wertz and Fletcher, 1988). Nonetheless, the degree of concordance between publicly espoused beliefs and actual practices is unknown, and some evidence (Fraser, 1979; Karp, 1983) suggests that under some circumstances divergence does occur.

[1]This essay first appeared as Kessler S (1992) Psychological aspects of genetic counseling. VII. Thoughts on directiveness. *Journal of Genetic Counseling* 1:9–17. Reprinted with kind permission of the publisher, Kluwer Academic/Human Sciences Press.

In genetic counseling, directiveness and nondirectiveness are taken to mean, respectively, the rendering or withholding of direct advice, generally about reproduction and abortion. Some genetic counselors frame the issue solely in terms of responses to "What would you do" questions. However, in my opinion, this is too narrow a conceptualization. Directiveness implies more; there is an attempt on the part of the counselor to persuade the counselee to pursue a specific course of action.

In rendering advice or informing a counselee as to what their personal choice might be in a given situation, the counselor overtly attempts to shape and influence the counselee's behavior. However, directiveness may be applied in more subtle or covert ways. For example, in providing genetic education, the counselor simultaneously may transmit direct and indirect attitudes, suggestions, value judgments, preferences, and directives simply by spending more time on one option rather than another or by expending slightly greater energy and enthusiasm on option A rather than option B. Just by focusing the counselee's attention on potential risks, genetic and otherwise, or on the consequences of genetic disease, the counselor communicates more than objective, neutral information. When the counselor tends to focus on the down side of a neural tube defect or Down syndrome rather than on the positive aspects or achievements of affected persons, it would not be unreasonable for the counselees to infer that they are being directed to avoid such disorders.

Because of the many covert ways of being directive, it should not be assumed that not answering questions as, "What would you do in my place?" establishes that one is being nondirective. Clever, efficacious directiveness, as anyone who has done hypnotic trance work knows, may be accomplished indirectly, through metaphor, story telling, and other subtle procedures. One does not have to answer "What would you do" questions to be directive.

In general, one does not have to answer a question to answer a question. An outstanding example of this was how CNN's Peter Arnett fielded questions under tight Iraqi censorship during the recent Gulf War. When asked about the presence of military vehicles on the road to the city of Basra, he replied, "There is a lot of traffic on the road and little of it is civilian." When asked about the deliberate placement of military hardware in the midst of civilian population centers, he replied, "If I answered that question I would be cut off the air." The questions were not answered and yet they were.

One might think that directiveness and nondirectiveness are polar opposites on a single dimension. I would like to suggest that they are not. In fact, there are more similarities in the two approaches than meets the eye. Both are counseling strategies in which an attempt is made to influence the counselee. In other words, both are forms of persuasion. In the case of directiveness, the counselor wishes to influence the counselee's behavior, whereas in the case of nondirectiveness, the counselor attempts to influence the way the counselee thinks about a specific problem. This, in turn, may ultimately also influence the counselee's behavior.

In nondirective counseling, the counselor tries to persuade the counselees to think that they have the capacity and ability to make and carry out their own decisions. In some ways, it is a technique in which the illusion is created that the counselees have control over their situation. Thus, the emphasis in nondirective counseling tends to be on the enhancement of the counselee's self-determining capacities.

In directiveness, there is a tendency to focus on the ideal choice or decision (either for society or for the individual). By being directive, the counselor attempts to create the illusion that he or she has taken responsibility for the counselees' actions and decisions, and since he or she is an authority, the directive carries the weight of the counselor's expertise.

A major difference between the two approaches is that the directive counselor may be more aware of his or her strategy and thus may be perceived as being more authentic in the counseling. Nondirective counselors either tend to deny that they are attempting to influence the counselee or are oblivious of making such attempts. As Haley (1963) and others point out, the strategy of influencing while one is denying one is doing so can be a powerfully persuasive tool in the counseling or therapeutic setting.

Viewed as counseling strategies, directive and nondirective approaches might be seen in a more positive, less conflicting light. There are times for one strategy and times for the other. I have always found that nondirective approaches are best to illuminate the direction of the counselees' thinking, their needs and wishes. Once these are clear, directive counseling that confirms the counselees' direction is often helpful to them.

What is needed is greater flexibility rather than dogmatism in genetic counseling practices. But such flexibility requires flexible counseling skills.

Discussions of directiveness often neglect to consider the level and quality of the interview skills of counselors. Direct questions posed to counselors or therapists are common occurrences in the personal counseling situation. These questions might be for direct advice ("What should I do?"), for opinions about one matter or another ("What do you think about . . ."), personal information about the counselor ("Are you married?"), etc. Experienced counselors learn to handle such questions adroitly, generally without ever answering them. This is often done by one of at least three different means. First, one can simply ignore direct questions and proceed as if the question was not asked. Second, one might respond using Peter Arnett-like answers, as discussed above. Third, one might redirect attention to a process issue. For example, a youngish-looking genetic counselor intern, working frequently with couples older than herself tended to be asked if she had children. In the course of supervision I asked her, "Why do you think they are asking you that question?" In discussing the matter she was able to see that it was irrelevant to the counselees whether or not she had progeny. What was relevant was their concern about whether she could understand their situation and help them. This led her to handle such questions by responding, "I'm wondering if you are concerned about whether or not I can understand what you are going through?" This answer to the counselees' question was far more empathic, satisfactory, and to the point than the number of children she had or did not have.

THE ARGUMENT FOR DIRECTIVENESS

A major argument for directiveness in genetic counseling has been that counselees want and expect such counseling from professionals. For example, Czeizel et al. (1981) state that their "counselees said they needed 'more help,' and asked for our advice too." Also, reports of directive counseling in Japan (Fujita, 1979), Romania (Christodorescu, 1980), and Switzerland (Klein and Wyss, 1977) are based on assumptions of consumer desire and sociocultural support for such counseling. However, data demonstrating such consumer desire are not there and one wonders whether or not in certain circumstances counselees have much choice in the matter.

In the United States, Lubs (1979) found that 62% of individuals with a family history of X-linked disorders thought a counselor should only present alternatives and not recommend a course of action around family planning; only 27% thought that direct advice was appropriate. These data seem strongly supportive of an overall nondirective counseling strategy, at least for U.S. populations.

Advocates of directiveness in genetic counseling sometimes argue that counselees cannot assess adequately the intricacies of scientific and technological information, thus they require the counselor's active intervention. The first part of this assumption is probably correct. But, not being able to assess information in the way that counselors do does not stop reproductive decision making under genetic risk. Considerable evidence points to the fact that the majority of counselees have already reached a decision about reproduction before they come for genetic counseling (Sissine et al., 1981; Wertz et al., 1984; Sorenson et al., 1987; Swerts, 1987). This suggests that one may not need to make a thorough assessment of all known knowledge before making an adequate or even optimum decision. If we did, almost any life decision would be nearly impossible.

A provocative argument for directiveness has been made by Pauker and Pauker (1979) who write that the "classic, nondirective model of genetic counseling . . . provides the consultants with information about risks, information, which the consultants must recall and combine with their own values to arrive at a decision. This frustrating process often results in the inevitable questions, 'Yes, Doctor, but what would you do?' or 'What do most people do at my age?' "

These investigators offer, instead, to obtain estimates of relative values of various outcomes from the counselee and then tell the counselee, via "explicit guidance," what decision logic dictates they make. This is not the place to describe and critique their model of decision making. Suffice it to say, their model does not work as well as they would like it to because, apparently, the parts do not add up to the whole and counselees frequently do not make the decisions the model suggests they ought to make.

The Paukers' statement warrants closer examination. First of all, their description of nondirective counseling, even in its classic form, may not be a fair portrayal. Second, on what basis do they say that nondirective counseling is frustrating? What is the evidence to support this assertion? I do not doubt that counselees might feel frustrated if a genetic counselor provided counseling in the way they describe. But, where are the supportive data? Third, what is the basis for their assertion that nondirective counseling often leads to "What would you do" questions? Again, what is the evidence?

I raise these questions not as criticism of the Paukers' model but as a way of exposing the areas of research begging for investigation. To my knowledge, no one has compared directive and nondirective genetic counseling in a meaningful way. Also, given the assumptions and all the ballyhoo about the "What would you do" questions, it is surprising that no one has documented how often these questions are actually asked in the genetic counseling arena. It may turn out that instances of requests for advice may be rare, in which case the Paukers' argument for directiveness would be undercut. Also, do certain counselors face these questions more frequently than others do? Should this turn out to be the case, it might suggest that the counselor may be saying or doing something that evokes these questions. One can easily imagine that counselors who are especially unclear in their discussions of etiology or risks, etc. or who are perceived as overly authoritative, authoritarian, or intimidating may be asked "What would you do" questions more frequently than counselors who have different styles. If this turns out to be the case, it would suggest that such questions are more a function of (and statement about) the counselor–counselee relationship than of a need for direction.

Bell (1990) has recently argued for more directiveness in genetic counseling. She points out that sometimes a strict adherence to a nondirective stance could leave the counselee hanging out on a limb (whatever that means). Bell believes that counselors should, when asked, share not only what decision they might make, but their personal decision-making processes as well. She also introduces a new twist to her argument, namely, that the sharing of internal process is a more "pliable" and female way of doing things, in which the "agony of decision . . . [is] shared."[2] It is unclear why or how the counselor's internal processes would be helpful to the counselee. It is likely that the counselor does not share the same life space, life history, and life dilemmas as the latter. The counselor may never have been married or pregnant or had an abortion. Also, imagine for a moment that the counselor is no clearer than the counselee in his or her own internal process regarding the decision the latter faces. In what way would the sharing of the counselor's confusion and uncertainty be helpful to imagine, for a moment that the counselor is no clearer than the counselee in counselee? This does not mean that the counselor may not be able to put himself or herself in the counselee's shoes and provide empathic assistance and, for that matter, help the counselee reach their own decision. However, no amount of empathy can replace the fact that the counselee has to make and live with their decision. The counselor does not share in the economic, social, and psychological consequences of a counselee's decision and so long as that is true how can the former ever honestly share in the "agony of decision."

Also, sharing one's internal processes of thoughts and feelings has a different meaning when a professional–client relationship is involved than, let us say, when two friends with a long-standing relationship of give and take get together socially. Presumably, in the latter instance, there is sufficient mutual trust to allow the sharing of internal processes of thoughts and feelings. Such trust comes from intimacy. In the professional–client relationship, on the other hand, such mutual trust would be desirable, and in long-term psychotherapy it sometimes becomes a possibility. In the short-term interactions of genetic counseling such trust is neither likely nor necessary.

---

[2]In a survey of genetic counselors carried out by Wertz and Fletcher (1988), it was found that male counselors were more likely than female counselors to say that they would provide directive counseling. In fact, all that is necessary in successful genetic counseling is unilateral trust of the counselee in the counselor.

RESEARCH ON DIRECTIVENESS/NONDIRECTIVENESS

In the course of other research, some preliminary light has been shed on the issue of directiveness in genetic counseling. For example, if genetic counselees want direct advice, one might expect that they would follow the advice they receive. What is the evidence that they do? Several studies bear on this question. In Hungary, before the present political liberalization, genetic counseling was (and may still be) directive. Czeizel et al. (1981) studied women who were either advised for or against pregnancy on the basis of their genetic risks. These investigators found that among counselees with high genetic risks (25–50%), 61% were "deterred" from a pregnancy. About one-third of the latter women were pregnant at the time of the counseling and had abortions. Because precounseling reproductive intentions were not studied, it is unclear whether or not the counseling influenced counselees to terminate or avoid pregnancies. What is noteworthy is that even under social and political conditions where directiveness is expected, nearly 40% of counselees with high genetic risks did not take the counselor's advice. In Romania, Christodorescu (1980) found that little change in precounseling reproductive intentions occurred after directive counseling. One can only conclude at this point that the effectiveness of directive genetic counseling has not been proven.

Another glimmer of light comes from studies of nondirective counseling. Lubs (1979) found that despite counseling said to be nondirective, about 9% of individuals faced with a genetic disorder perceived the genetic counselor as being directive. Shiloh and Saxe (1989) asked counselees after genetic counseling about their perceptions of counselor neutrality. Apparently, the six counselors were all U.S. physicians. These investigators found that only 42.5% of counselees perceived their counselor as neutral, whereas 32.9% and 24.7% of counselees, respectively, thought their counselors had given them direct and indirect advice about reproduction (Shiloh, personal communication). Unfortunately, the issue of directiveness was not the central focus of the Shiloh and Saxe study. Thus, the critical perceptions of the counselors about their own counseling were not obtained. Nonetheless, the study raises interesting questions. If the counselors' perceptions about their counseling differ significantly from those of the counselees, what would account for these differences? It should be noted that differences in perceptions between counselors and counselees about other central issues of genetic counseling have been shown by Wertz et al. (1988). For example, they found that in only 26% of sessions were both counselor and counselee aware of the major topic the other wished to discuss.

Future research may want to probe the questions of directiveness or nondirectiveness in genetic counseling. We need to know the extent to which counseling philosophy and practice intersect. Does what genetic counselors say they do relate to what they actually do in the course of counseling? Study of the process of genetic counseling may be the only way to answer this question and to clarify the operational differences and similarities between directiveness and nondirectiveness.

Also, it would be intriguing to ascertain if the individuals or couples who are still undecided about reproduction before counseling are the ones most likely to ask the counselor for advice. If it turns out that "What would you do" questions are (also) asked by individuals who have already made up their minds about reproduction, etc. before counseling, it would suggest that the literal interpretation of such questions might be off the mark. In reviewing the research on the effectiveness of genetic counseling, one is struck by how little influence such counseling has in changing precounseling reproductive plans (Kessler, 1989). Apparently, the variables on which counselors place high value, especially risk figures, often do not seem to play the role in the decisions of counselees that counselors think they should (Frets et al., 1990). Counselors strongly motivated by a directive bent might say that this fact argues for greater directiveness in the genetic counseling situation. Some counselors have the fantasy and wish that if they could only exert their personal power of persuasion, others would begin to see the world the way they do. This may be true, but it might also reflect an underlying sense of impotence or frustration about the ways things are. Perhaps, genetic counselors need to learn what others engaged in personal counseling and psychotherapy have had to resign themselves to and that is that we are not very powerful when it comes to changing the behavior of others. We do have some small successes generally for which both counselor and counselee have to work hard. But, on the whole, we are limited and it is a very humbling realization.

REFERENCES

Antley RM (1979) The genetic counselor as facilitator of the counselee's decision process. Birth Defects: Original Article Series 15(2):137–168.

Bell NK (1990) Medical ethicist responds to issue of non-directiveness in genetic counseling setting. Perspect Gen Counsel 12(4):5.

Christodorescu D (1980) Genetic counselling for neurological and psychic diseases. 1. Data on counsellees and their pre- and post-counselling family planning. Rev Roum Med Neural Psychiat 18:269–279.

Czeizel A, Metneki J, Osztovics M (1981) Evaluation of information-guidance genetic counselling. J Med Genet 18:91–98.

Fraser FC (1979) Degree of directiveness. In: Lubs HA, de la Cruz F (eds). Genetic Counseling. New York: Raven Press, pp 579–581.

Frets PG, Duivenvoorden HJ, Verhage F, Niermeijer MF, van den Berge SMM, Galjaard H (1990) Factors influencing the reproductive decision after genetic counseling. Am J Med Genet 35:496–502.

Fujita N (1979) Genetic counselling: follow-up study. Metab Pediat Ophthal 3:237–246.

Haley J (1963) Strategies in Psychotherapy. New York: Grune & Stratton.

Karp LE (1983) Genetic drift: the terrible question. Am J Med Genet 14:1–4.

Kessler S (1989) Psychological aspects of genetic counseling. VI. A critical review of the literature dealing with education and reproduction. Am J Med Genet 34:340–353.

Klein D, Wyss D (1977) Retrospective and follow up study of approximately 1000 genetic consultations. J Genet Hum 25:47–57.

Lubs ML (1979) Does genetic counseling influence risk attitudes and decision making? Birth Defects: Original Article Series 15(5C):355–367.

Pauker SP, Pauker SG (1979) The amniocentesis decision: an explicit guide for parents. Birth Defects: Original Article Series 5(5C):289–324.

Shiloh S, Saxe L (1989) Perception of risk in genetic counseling. Psychol Health 3:45–61.

Sissine FJ, Rosser L, Steele MW, Marchese S, Garver KL, Berman N (1981) Statistical analysis of genetic counseling impacts. Eval Rev 5:745–757.

Sorenson JR, Scotch NA, Swazcy JP, Wertz DC, Heeren TC (1987) Reproductive plans of genetic counseling clients not eligible for prenatal diagnosis. Am J Med Genet 28:345–352.

Swerts A (1987) Impact of genetic counseling and prenatal diagnosis for Down syndrome and neural tube defects. Birth Defects: Original Article Series 23(2):61–83.

Wertz DC, Fletcher JC (1988) Attitudes of genetic counselors: a multinational survey. Am J Hum Genet 42:592–600.

Wertz DC, Sorenson JR, Heeren TC (1984) Genetic counseling and reproductive uncertainty. Am J Med Genet 18:79–88.

Wertz DC, Sorenson JR, Heeren TC (1988) Communication in health professional–lay encounters: how often does each party know what the other wants to discuss. In: Ruben BD (ed). Information and Behavior, Vol 2. New Brunswick, NJ: Transaction Books, pp 329–342.

12

Nondirectiveness Revisited[1]

INTRODUCTION

It is unclear who first introduced the term *nondirectiveness* (ND) into the genetic counseling literature. It is likely that Sheldon Reed, who had earlier coined the term *genetic counseling* (Reed, 1949), may have been instrumental in this regard. By the early 1960s, Reed (1964, 1974) borrowed the concepts directiveness and ND from the field of psychotherapy and associated them, respectively, with the giving and withholding of advice. In contrasting the methods of psychiatry and genetic counseling, he stated, "[T]he geneticist cannot indulge in directives" (Reed, 1964). During this period, others addressed the same issue without using the term *nondirective*. Lynch (1969), for example, wrote:

> The counselor must never make decisions for the (client) regarding marriage, children, and other important personal issues. These decisions are the (client's) responsibility and only (the client) should exercise this right.

By the mid-1970s, these terms were firmly entrenched in the genetic counseling literature, although some medical geneticists had their doubts about pursuing a nondirective course. Porter (1979), for example, in the halcyon period before HMOs, managed care, and the contemporary erosion of physician authority, wrote:

> [T]he neutrality of the counselor . . . is unusual in medical practice, and is a difficult attitude for many physicians to adopt. . . . With prolonged experience and with more

[1]This essay first appeared as Kessler S (1997) Psychological aspects of genetic counseling. XI. Nondirectiveness revisited. *American Journal of Medical Genetics* 72:164–171. Reprinted with kind permission of the publisher, John Wiley and Sons.

physicians providing genetic counseling, we may expect a change to the more traditional doctor–patient relationship.

Nonetheless, the 1970s saw a gathering momentum among geneticists toward a nondirective approach. By the mid-1980s, surveys of medical geneticists around the world showed an overwhelming endorsement of ND in genetic counseling (Wertz and Fletcher, 1988). More recently, a nondirective approach was strongly endorsed by Baumiller et al. (1996) in their code of ethical principles for professionals in genetic services.

Besides the anti-eugenics conviction of many geneticists (Ludmerer, 1972; Porter, 1979; Fine, 1993) and the already changing nature of medical practice, the shift in thinking toward ND was influenced by the growing consumerism movement. There was an increased awareness among geneticists that they often dealt with life problems and decisions about which they had no greater expertise than anyone else. Last, but not least, there was the growing number of nonphysician professional women entering the field of genetic counseling. Women, more than men, are likely to be nondirective (Wertz, 1994).

Like most concepts transposed from one field to another, something often gets lost in translation. Thus, the focus or emphasis on whether or not advice was given tended to lead to a neglect of other important aspects of what was involved in directiveness and ND. For example, almost totally neglected were the counseling techniques associated with ND, which provided the means by which the ideal of ND could be achieved. It is not surprising then to read frequent complaints in the genetic counseling literature about the difficulty—some say impossibility—of achieving ND. The *how* of ND was misplaced in transposing this concept to genetic counseling.

In this paper, I would like to examine the psychological meaning of ND and show how a fuller understanding of it might be applied to the practice of genetic counseling. First, let us examine directiveness to see what light might be shed on ND.

DIRECTIVENESS

Attempts to influence us are ubiquitous. All the social institutions to which we are exposed (e.g., the family, churches and other religious institutions, school, political and professional groups, advertisers, and merchants) all try to influence our attitudes and behavior and we expect them to. In all of these attempts, the element of individual choice or autonomy is not compromised, especially as we approach and enter adulthood. We can choose which language to study to fulfill our requirements in school, which automobile to buy, which political party to vote for, which brand of toothpaste to purchase, and which social causes to support. In this regard, our autonomy and our ability to accept reject suggestions and other attempts to influence our behavior remain relatively intact.

However, there is a form of persuasive communication in which our ability to choose and our individuality and autonomy are suppressed. In such situations, the individual is unaware that the other party has a hidden agenda and that *that* agenda is to systematically and deliberately gain control over our attitudes and behavior.

By limiting access to information and contact with others with differing viewpoints, and by creating a sense of powerlessness and fear, our usual behavior can be changed and new behavior substituted so that we act in ways we would not otherwise have chosen. No one is immune to this process. Psychologists call this *persuasive* coercion, or as it is more commonly known, mind control or brain washing. Our knowledge of such techniques comes from several sources, but most recently from the study of the way cults actively recruit and incorporate new members and keep them in the fold (Singer, 1995).

Directiveness in genetic counseling needs to be thought of as a form of persuasive coercion. Like all such techniques, one or more of the following elements exist: deception, threat, or coercion.

I am being directive if I advertise in the telephone yellow pages that I am a provider of abortion services (as some pro-life groups have done), and recruit unsuspecting women seeking to terminate a pregnancy; if I subject them to intense efforts, such as showing graphic videotapes of fetuses being torn apart or supposedly writhing in pain in utero, efforts all designed to convince them to continue the pregnancy; if I tell them that what they have in mind is evil and sinful, that they will be punished for their actions; if physically, I won't let them leave until they promise to reconsider or change their decision. I have employed deception and I have used threatening and coercive procedures to change the women's attitudes and behavior.

One is also being directive when a salient option is purposely withheld from clients in order to shape (or coerce) their decision in a specific direction. If a professional deliberately spends considerable time discussing the negative aspects of trisomy 21 and gives very little time to any positive ones, directiveness is clearly involved. However, sometimes out of inattention, carelessness, thoughtlessness, or inadequate teaching or counseling skills, professionals may *unwittingly* omit or overemphasize one option over another. Clients might interpret such professional behavior as an imperative to act in a given direction, a mindset no different from that induced by deliberate coercion.[2] I tend to see these situations as "phenocopies" of directiveness arising as the result of inadequacies in the professional's training and ability to apply counseling procedures.

In the genetic counseling literature, ND is often formulated as the absence of directiveness as if the two concepts were mutually exclusive. This I believe is a mistake. There is a vast gray area between directiveness, with its techniques of coercion (Milunsky, 1975; Antley, 1979), and ND. Much of what occurs in genetic counseling falls into this gray zone. By themselves disparate behaviors, such as giving directions, conveying information, making health-promoting suggestions, giving "bad" news, giving advice, and expressing one's biases, are neither directive nor nondirective. With the introduction of deception and coercive techniques, these activities become directive.

Ignoring coercion as the defining issue in directiveness leads to a position in which almost any action or utterance in genetic counseling could be interpreted as

[2] I thank Dr. Dorothy Wertz for bringing this to my attention.

directiveness. The result is an unrealistic lumping together of all forms of advice, directions, suggestions and recommendations, helpful or not, coercive and noncoercive, into a single, undifferentiated hodgepodge. A recent study (Michie et al., 1997) illustrates this point. Not one of the examples they give as being directive show any evidence of coercion, threat, or deception. In fact, depending on the counseling context, some of their examples might just as easily be considered as nondirective or just neutral.

Giving advice requires comment because it often serves, mistakenly in my opinion, as the focal point in the genetic counseling literature to differentiate directiveness and ND. First, there are ways to provide advice in a nondirective way (see below). Second, advice can be given in a noncoercive way, which does not compromise client's ability to choose or does not undermine their autonomy. Third, noncoercive professional advice does not seem to carry the weight or authority or influence it once did in the past. Many clients resist, distort, or ignore advice that does not match their preconceived ideas of risks and precounseling decisions (see Kessler (1989) for a review of the literature).

Nondirectiveness

Nondirectiveness owes its origin to psychoanalysis and psychodynamic therapy. The original concept described a procedure in which the analyst or therapist deliberately held back from interfering with the verbal production of the patient in order to encourage free association. In the 1930s and early 1940s, Carl Rogers (1942) appropriated the term ND to describe his personal approach to psychotherapy, which, similar to the psychodynamic tradition, gave clients the leeway to set the agenda, pace, and direction of their therapy. In the 1950s, for political reasons more than anything else, he renamed his system "client-centered therapy" (Rogers, 1951), in order to emphasize the fact that he was rejecting the medical model of treating psychological problems.

Placing the full control of the agenda, pacing, and direction of treatment in the hands of the client is, I believe, applicable only to psychotherapy and not genetic counseling. Because of the relatively short duration of professional–client contact and other factors (Kessler, 1997a), such procedures are really not a viable option. Thus, in this regard, genetic counseling is neither Rogerian nor client centered. By and large, attempts to apply these terms to genetic counseling are, in my view, misguided.

On the other hand, since the beginning, there has been a second aspect of nondirective methods that practitioners recognized, namely their ability to promote the autonomous functioning of the client. This aspect of ND is clearly applicable to genetic counseling and I offer it as a definition: *ND describes procedures aimed at promoting the autonomy* and *self-directedness of the client*.

Note that much more than withholding or not giving advice is involved. It is possible to withhold advice and yet not be nondirective, just as it is possible to give advice and remain nondirective. The secret in the latter case is *how* the advice is given.

Let us examine two apparently contrasting excerpts (in both instances the professional (P) is a male medical geneticist; W = woman; M = man).

Example 1

In the first excerpt, a couple has had a previous pregnancy in which a trisomy was found (based on Fraser, 1979):

> P: [*Explains the low recurrence risk and the possibility of amniocentesis.*]
>
> W: I want it.
>
> M: I don't believe in abortion. Well, what are we going to do?
>
> [*Further discussion ensues.*]
>
> M: Well, what do we do?
>
> P: Well it's not my problem. I am not you. You'll have to come to some resolution with your conscience and work it out with your wife. [More discussion ensues.]
>
> W: What would you do if you had the trisomy child?
>
> P: Well, one can never say what they actually would do in a situation. But I think I would be willing to take advantage of these means and be sure I don't have a recurrence.

The professional here is dealing with a couple who seems to disagree about whether or not to have an amniocentesis (see too a comparable analysis of this same excerpt by Wolff and Jung (1995)). Unfortunately, he neither acknowledges the disagreement nor explores what is at stake here, two very basic counseling strategies. For example, it is unclear whether or not M objects to having the amniocentesis. Is his focus only on abortion? The limits of his objection are not made explicit. Is he willing to go along with W if she insists? Would he leave the relationship if she went ahead with the amniocentesis or with an abortion? These implications are not made known at this point, and may have an impact on the subsequent course of the session.

After M asks for advice a second time, the professional distances himself and rebuffs him ("Well it's not my problem. I am not you."). Of course, we do not have information about the inner state of the professional at this point. His statements could easily be interpreted by M as a form of rejection and as an expression of annoyance for being placed in the position of "having" to give advice. Finally, the professional relents. With some qualification, he takes sides with W against M and gives advice without establishing the context for it or the possible fallout of taking sides.

Fraser (1979) believes that this is directive counseling. However, there is no effort to coerce the couple and there is certainly no deception involved. Thus, I see no evidence of directiveness. However, several details stand out. An obvious one is the professional's initial ambivalence about giving advice, which seems to give way as he becomes caught up in the clients' conflict(s). His strategy to disengage from the conflict is to take sides, which is not the best counseling procedure. As the professional seems to experience and report the exchange with W and M, he is pressured into being directive, thus implying that it was the clients' responsibility that advice had to be given.[3] Also, although many details of the actual session are not available, the pro-

---

[3]This very argument is advanced by the President's Commission (1983), which essentially places the onus of directiveness on the clients for what in reality may be inadequacies in counseling skills among professionals.

fessional seems uncomfortable in the counseling role and has difficulty sustaining a nondirective course.

Example 2

In the second example, a woman who has had a previous child (deceased) with a neural tube defect is speaking:

> W: Do most people go ahead and have this [amnio] in our situation?
>
> P: Do most people? I can't answer. What do you mean by "most"? By far the largest group of couples who come for amniocentesis are women of age 35 or above. [*He goes on to distinguish between most women and most women referred to the clinic.*]
>
> W: Do these things happen just because, I mean, for no reason?
>
> P: [*sarcastically*] There's nothing that has no reason. . . . [*Explains genetic mechanisms again.*]
>
> W: But, would you advise . . . to have it?
>
> P: I, that's not my decision to make. All I can tell you what the—
>
> W: [*interrupts*] Yeah, but if it were your sister sitting there, and she, I—
>
> P: [*interrupts*] I wouldn't be able to advise my sister on what to do.

Here the professional sidesteps the client's questions and withholds advice. Is he being nondirective? I think not. Notice how he deals with the client. He shows difficulties in relatively simple counseling procedures (some of which parallel those the professional in the previous example had). First, he shows no evidence that he understands what is on the client's mind. Second, he does not explore the dilemmas the client may have that impede her decision making. In fact, he shows little interest at all in the client's thinking. Third, he shows or expresses absolutely no empathy toward her. He seems to miss the fact that she is desperate to hear that she was not responsible for her previous child's problems and she needs his reassurance in this regard. Fourth, he says things that are patently unbelievable, particularly about how he might deal with his hypothetical sister. Fifth, he is not helpful to the client. He gives no assistance on possible alternative ways of thinking about her problems or decisions. Lastly, he distances himself from and finally becomes demeaning and nasty toward her. In short, he does not promote the autonomy and self-directedness of the client. Thus, he is not being nondirective even though he has not given advice.

What we have here is a professional who may be extremely competent in everything else he does. He may be a very good diagnostician and a competent medical geneticist. However, he does not know the basic rudiments of counseling techniques. In short, this is an example of unskillful, incompetent counseling. In my mind, this is the kernel of the so-called problem many genetic counselors seem to have with ND.

I suggest that one cannot achieve ND without a minimum of basic counseling skills. I do not mean the kind of skills one might need to help clients in their decision making or to change their personalities; I am referring to basic Counseling 101 skills.

The persisting problems of ND arise largely from inadequacies in applying simple, basic counseling procedures.

As I read the genetic counseling literature I cannot help but be struck by the frequency with which the statement is made that ND is unachievable. What I hear in this perpetual repetition is a public confession that counselors have either inadequate counseling skills or no confidence in the skills they do have. Also, it is a prediction of failure with self-fulfilling consequences.

How would an experienced counselor with a nondirective bent go about dealing with the clients in the above examples? Let us begin with the couple from Example 1.

Example 3

An experienced counselor would probably have dealt with the disagreement between the couple as follows:

W: I want it [the amnio]—

M: I don't believe in abortion.

P: Correct me if I'm wrong but [*to W*] you seem to want the amnio procedure. I'm not sure how you [*to M*] feel about it?

The strategy here would have been to try to separate the issue of having an amniocentesis from that of having an abortion, thus parceling out the problem into more manageable chunks. Later in the session when M asks again:

M: Well, what are we going to do?

P: I'm not sure I know what you mean when you say you don't *believe* in abortion?

The strategy at this point would have been to obtain clarification of the client's belief system(s) (i.e., no abortion ever; abortion sometimes, etc.). It would also be important to establish how flexible or rigid M's belief system is (i.e., would he leave his wife if she decided to have an abortion?). An alternative strategy would have been:

M: Well, what are we going to do?

P: When you ask me, "What are we to do?" what do you see as the problem?

That question might have elicited important information for the professional. M might have said that he wants the latter to be the judge as to who had the "correct" position. The professional might then have had an opportunity to tell the clients that he was not a judge, only a counselor, and that whatever advice he could give would require that he take sides, and since it was more important that he retain the confidence of both of them, that was not what he wanted to do. He might then have turned to them and asked how they resolve differences of opinion in other circumstances. He might then have used that as a model of how they might resolve the present problem.

In sum, there were multiple, simple means the professional might have used to remain neutral and help the couple reach a satisfactory decision without resorting to advice giving.

Example 4

In Example 2, the following might have been said:

W: Do these things happen just because, I mean, for no reason?

P: Yes, those things happen right at conception, right from the beginning and we don't know or understand why. But, one thing's for sure; you definitely didn't make it happen in your last pregnancy.

The professional here attempts to relieve the client's sense of responsibility for having caused the initial problem. The approach shows respect for her question and for her unstated concerns.

W: What would you advise your sister?

P: I suppose if my sister had turned to me for advice I would ask her the same questions I would ask you. How would she feel if she didn't have the amnio and then had a child with a genetic problem? Would she be able to live with it and with herself, or would she berate herself for the rest of her life? Also, I would ask her what she might do if she had the amnio and we found that the fetus had a genetic problem? What would she do then? How do *you* feel about these issues?

Here the professional provides a framework by which the client might think through the problem facing her and arrive at her own decision. By treating the client in the same way the professional might treat his sister, notice how the emotional distance between professional and client is narrowed as if to give the message that we are both human beings struggling together to find some solutions. Contrast this with the first excerpt (Example 1) in which the professional says things that promote a psychological chasm between himself and the clients.

Following are some further examples of how experienced counselors go about being nondirective.

Example 5

This is a reply to the question, "What would you do in my place?"

P: I really don't know what I'd do in your place, but I can tell you how I might think about it. There's part of me that would be saying I want another child and I want it to be healthy and another part that's afraid that if I did have a child I would have one with a problem and that's not what I want. So I guess I would have to ask myself am I ready and willing to take the risk to have a child knowing that there are no guarantees in life. What are your thoughts about that?

As in the previous example, the professional here provides a suggested framework the clients might use to think through their problem or dilemma so that they might arrive at their own solution. The underlying message is also one in which the professional strongly implies that he has confidence in the clients' ability to reach their own decision.

Example 6

The following is an alternative approach to the same question, "What would you do in my place?"

> P: Look, I'm just another human being like you and I have the same concerns and anxieties you might have. It wouldn't be any easier for me to make the decision you're facing than it is for you. I would discuss it with my mate and find out how he (she) feels about this situation and see if we're on the same wavelength or not. If we are, that's fine. If not, I would try to find some compromise or common ground and if necessary get outside help. Somewhere inside of me I know what's best for me just like somewhere inside of you, you know what's best for you. Let's see if I can help you find that place in yourself so that you can do what feels right for you. What do you think?

Contrast the above approach to what the professional said to his clients in Example 1. In the approach here, the professional identifies with the clients' humanity and with their dilemma. There is a profound psychological impact when clients feel that the professional with whom they are dealing can identify with and understand their feelings and confusions, respect them despite their possibly perceived failings, and help them by giving them a way of thinking about their problem.

Example 7

The following is a nondirective approach to the question, "What do most people do in our situation"?:

> P: Most people go through the same kind of process you're going through. They have to face the same dilemmas and choices you do and each person, each couple, has to make a decision that feels right for them, a decision they can live with. I wish that decisions like this were easier to make, but usually for most couples they're not. Some people decide to go one way and some decide just the opposite. In the end you have to make a decision that fits your personal needs and goals and feels best for you. Any way I can help you make that decision I'll sure try. What are your thoughts?

The professional here expresses empathy for the clients' dilemma and tells them that they are part of the normative population in their efforts to find a satisfactory solution. Again, he offers to help them in their struggle, but no advice is given.

ADVICE-GIVING

Earlier on it was suggested that one might give advice and remain nondirective. The following examples (8–11) address that point:

Example 8

P: Would you mind if I made a suggestion to you? [*The professional waits for permission to continue.*] *I might be misreading the situation*, but it *seems* to me that you've been through a lot and maybe now's not the time to have a baby. What do you think?

Example 9

P: Joan, I've known you for quite a while now and I think I have a good idea of what you're thinking. Of course, *I could be wrong*, but it *seems* to me that when you're ready you might consider the possibility of another child. What are your thoughts?

Example 10

P: *I might be off base*, and remember *I don't know you as well as you know yourselves*, but it *seems* to me that there may be advantages in taking this test. [*Outline one or two advantages.*] What are your thoughts?

Example 11

P: Here's a suggestion. Take it for what it's worth, reject all or part of it if you want, because I could be way off base, you know the situation far better than I do, but I think perhaps . . . etc. etc. What do you think?

What makes the examples above nondirective is two things. First, the counselor presents the advice as a suggestion as if it were a possibility of action rather than a certainty in his mind. Notice too how the suggestions are worded, especially the words in italics, so as to deliberately emphasize the seeming tentativeness rather than the certainty of each situation and of the professional's thinking. This is a common nondirective strategy used to de-emphasize the professional's image as one based on authority (Kessler, 1997b).

Second, the professional gives the client permission, either implicitly or explicitly, to reject all or part of the advice being proffered. Such strategies protect and promote the clients' self-directedness and ability to make their own choice. Notice also how experienced counselors invariably turn back to the client for feedback immediately after giving the suggestion. This allows for timely corrections, modification, or additional input and underscores that the professional and client are working together toward a common goal.

Although nondirective counselors occasionally give advice, they do so judiciously and rarely because with experience they learn that there are major pitfalls in doing so. Often we do not always know what advice to give. Also, we cannot live other people's lives for them. When professionals give advice, which is subsequently rejected by clients, they risk jeopardizing the confidence the latter may have in them. Furthermore, unless advice concurs with the clients' thinking, it may make their decision making more difficult. Also, there is no strong evidence that clients follow the advice they receive.[4] Last, but by no means least, giving advice tends to gratify the ego needs of professionals more than those of clients. Psychologically, advice-giving helps one feel less helpless or more powerful in their professional role.

DISCUSSION

I have attempted to demonstrate here how the goal of ND is closely linked to counseling procedures. ND is more than withholding advice. It is a way of interacting and working with clients that aims to raise their self-esteem and leave them with greater control over their lives and decisions. Genetic counseling based on the provision of information (Hsia, 1979; President's Commission, 1983) is limited in achieving these goals. Information-giving may provide facts, but does not necessarily give clients a way of thinking about the information they receive. It also tends to emphasize the professional's authority and knowledge, factors that tend to foster psychological passivity in clients. Such passivity, in turn, interferes with their evaluative processes and self-directiveness and tends to increase their dependency on professional advice (Kessler, 1997a).

When clients come into contact with professionals, they place themselves in a disadvantaged position and, for some, the context is stacked against them (Clarke, 1991). Professionals have authority and knowledge that clients lack, and thus are in a relatively superior position. In addition, clients sometimes have unrealistic expectations of professionals and believe that the latter are always unbiased and have no self-interest. Directive professionals take advantage of such naivete and inexperience to promote their own agendas. Nondirective professionals actively adopt a strategy that, from the onset of the session, aims to restore the power balance between themselves and clients.

Thus, ND is an *active* strategy requiring quality counseling skills. ND does not happen by default or by not directing the client toward a particular decision or course of action. Just as professionals with a directive agenda actively direct or guide clients to a particular decision and course of action, so do nondirective professionals (Kessler, 1992). The difference is that the latter strive to guide clients to their *own* decision, not the one the professional might make or believe the client should make. ND is a way of thinking about the professional–client relationship in which at each step

---

[4]In some sociopolitical circumstances in which directive genetic counseling was the norm, as for example Communist-dominated Hungary, nearly 40% of counselees ignored the professional's advice (Czeizel et al., 1981).

of the way the professional attempts to evoke the client's competence and ability for self-direction.

The difficulties genetic counselors seem to have in dealing with direct questions, handling commonplace counseling issues, providing empathy and a way of thinking about problems (rather than giving advice), in combination with other problems, to be discussed below, all suggest the presence of major inadequacies in counseling training and skill. These deficiencies clearly need to be corrected if the field is to adhere to a nondirective philosophy.

Why genetic counselors seem to have trouble dealing with direct questions is puzzling and perhaps a way of thinking about the problem would be in order. When clients ask us for our advice, what do they want?[5] A nondirective approach would assume, among other things, that most clients have the ability to make their own decisions. Thus, nondirective professionals would infer that something beyond the literal was intended by the question. They might think to themselves, "After all, not all statements or all questions are meant to be understood literally." For example, when I ask clients, "What brought you to the clinic?" I do not want them to understand me literally and reply, "I came by bus." I want them to outline the problem about which they are concerned. In fact, when a client does answer seriously in such a concrete manner, I would begin to suspect the presence of neurological organicity. So, what lies behind the question?

The professional might then entertain some plausible possibilities, among which are:

1. It might be a way of asking for clarification of previously given information.
2. It carries a psychological message suggesting that clients experience the professional as being too detached and emotionally unconnected to them. Thus, their question may be an attempt to elicit a greater involvement of the professional's human side, as if to say, "Please, put yourself in my place and feel what I'm feeling—understand me." Rather than give advice, this realization might lead to a change in how they relate to clients.

Nondirective strategies require professionals to pay more attention to the strengths, accomplishments, and competencies that clients bring with them to genetic counseling. These need to be verbally acknowledged and bolstered throughout the session so that clients feel that the professional has confidence in their ability to make their own decisions. Most clients are already experienced decision-makers, and professionals need to draw on the intelligence, life experiences, and know-how they have used in the past to deal with current issues (Parsons and Atkinson, 1993).

Clients also need to be encouraged to talk more in the counseling session, because this gives them a sense that they have greater control over the situation. This is almost impossible if the professional uses up the available "air time" giving information. In general, clients receive far more information in genetic counseling than they can possibly absorb and integrate. Some of these difficulties might be

[5]Milunsky (1975) is close to the truth when he writes that such questions "may signal failure in counseling . . . [and that clients] are not interested in what the professional would do in like circumstances."

alleviated if professionals utilized alternative means of providing information, such as written formats and interactive technology, and then used the time together with clients more effectively as counselors.

Professionals need to learn how and when to reward clients and reinforce any effort toward autonomy and self-direction. This may mean that their need to be seen as authorities may have to be restrained in order to make room for the expression of the clients' autonomy and individuality.

Most important, professionals need to learn how to help clients think problems through, the skills exemplified in Examples 4–6 above. This is a view consistent with recommendations made by Brunger and Lippman (1995) and Kenen and Smith (1995). Teaching students that they only need to know how to be "good listeners" or how to be "supportive" in order to be genetic counselors are Pollyanna-ish ideas of what counseling is about. Such attitudes tend to reinforce their passivity and inhibit the acquisition of more effective, active skills.

Counselors are professionals who have acquired, and are in various stages of mastering, certain skills. These include keeping their personal feelings, thoughts, and opinions to themselves and sufficiently under control so that they do not intrude into their work. To the extent that it is humanly possible, they stay focused on the thoughts, feelings, and needs of their clients, not on their own.

Also, they have learned to identify and control their feelings of aggression (see Example 2 above) and competitiveness as well as their tendencies to be emotionally distant and self-absorbed, which often accompany such feelings. An example of how genetic counselors compete with clients occurs when the former say, "I will support any decision you make." This is often a subtle form of competition for the moral high ground or for power, in which the professional gives the client a subtle reminder that the professional still holds the greater power. This is a strategy I would strongly discourage. It may be sufficient to tell clients that you understand how they feel.

How does one acquire nondirective counseling skills? There are four traditional steps. First is self-knowledge. Here we invariably need outside help since we generally are blind to our faults and failings and generally distort our perceived strengths and limitations. I would strongly recommend a course of personal psychotherapy with a cognitive-behavioral slant as a way of identifying and changing the beliefs about self and others that impede our ability to be empathic and helpful as counselors.

Second is practical course work in counseling procedures in which we receive feedback and constructive criticism and are helped to acquire and practice basic skills.

Third is ongoing, regular postgraduate supervision and consultation. There are a number of "old-timers" in the field of genetic counseling who would be invaluable assets in this regard and could provide the needed support to working with genetic counselors.

Fourth is continuing education. A counselor is never a "finished" professional. I would strongly recommend that professional organizations sponsor workshops using resources from within the field itself in which professionals have an opportunity to hone their skills and learn new ways to approach old problems.

As far as ND is concerned, the message needs to be: It *is* attainable; all you need is a few basic skills, considerable good will, and kindness.

ACKNOWLEDGMENT

This article is based on a lecture given at the National Society of Genetic Counselors Annual Educational Conference, San Francisco, CA, on October 27, 1996, and is dedicated to the memory of Dr. Beverley R. Rollnick

REFERENCES

Antley RM (1979) Genetic Counseling: Facts, Values, and Norms. Birth Defects: Original Article Series 15(2):137–168.

Baumiller RC, Cunningham G, Fisher N, Fox L, Henderson M, Lebel R, McGrath G, Pelias MZ, Porter I, Seydel F, Wilson R (1996) Code of ethical principles for genetics professionals: an explication. Am J Med Genet 65:179–183.

Brunger F, Lippman A (1995) Resistance and adherence to the norms of genetic counseling. J Genet Counsel 4:151–167.

Clarke A (1991) Is non-directive counselling possible? Lancet 336:998–1001.

Czeizel A, Metnéki J, Osztóvics (1981) Evaluation of information-guidance genetic counselling. J Med Genet 18:91–98.

Fine BA (1993) The evolution of nondirectiveness in genetic counseling and implications of the human genome project. In: Bartels D, LeRoy BS, Kaplan A (eds). Prescribing Our Future: Ethical Challenges in Genetic Counseling. New York: Aldine de Gruyer, pp 101–117.

Fraser FC (1979) Degree of directiveness. In: Lubs HA, de la Cruz F (eds). Genetic Counseling. New York: Raven Press, pp 579–581.

Hsia YE (1979) Genetic Counseling: Facts, Values and Norms. Birth Defects: Original Article Series 15(2):169–186.

Kenen RH, Smith ACM (1995) Genetic counseling for the next 25 years: models for the future. J Genet Counsel 4:115–124.

Kessler S (1989) Psychological aspects of genetic counseling. VI. A critical review of the literature dealing with education and reproduction. Am J Med Genet 34:340–353.

Kessler S (1992) Psychological aspects of genetic counseling. VII. Thoughts on directiveness. J Genet Counsel 1:9–17.

Kessler S (1997a) Psychological aspects of genetic counseling. IX. Teaching and counseling. J Gen Counsel 6:287–296.

Kessler S (1997b) Psychological aspects of genetic counseling. X. Advanced counseling techniques. J Gen Counsel 6:379–392.

Ludmerer KM (1972) Genetics and American Society. Baltimore: Johns Hopkins University Press.

Lynch HT (1969) Dynamic Genetic Counseling for Clinicians. Springfield, IL: CC Thomas.

Milunsky A (1975) The Prevention of Genetic Disease and Mental Retardation. Philadelphia: W.B. Saunders.

Michie S, Bron F, Bobrow M, Marteau TM (1997) Nondirectiveness in genetic counseling: an empirical study. Am J Hum Genet 60:40–47.

Parsons E, Atkinson P (1993) Genetic risk and reproduction. Sociol Rev 41:679–706.

Porter IH (1979) Evolution of genetic counseling in America. In: Lubs HA, de la Cruz F (eds). Genetic Counseling. New York: Raven Press, pp 17–34.

President's Commission for the Study of Ethical Problems in Medicine and Biomedical and Behavioral Research (1983) Report on Screening and Counseling for Genetic Conditions. Washington, DC: Superintendent of Documents.

Reed SC (1949) Counseling in human genetics. Dight Institute Bull. No. 6. Minneapolis: University of Minnesota Press.

Reed SC (1964) Genetic counseling. In: Human Genetics in Public Health. Proceedings of Symposium on Human Genetics in Public Health. Minneapolis, MN, Aug. 9–11, 1964, pp 35–37.

Reed SC (1974) A short history of genetic counseling. Soc Biol 21:332–339.

Rogers CH (1942) Counseling and Psychotherapy: Newer Concepts in Practice. Boston: Houghton Mifflin.

Rogers CH (1951) Client-Centered Therapy: Its Current Practice, Implications and Theory. Boston: Houghton Mifflin.

Singer MT (1995) Cults in Our Midst. San Francisco: Jossey-Bass.

Wertz DC (1994) Provider gender and moral reasoning: the politics of an Ethics of Care. J Genet Counsel 3:95–112.

Wertz DC, Fletcher JC (1988) Attitudes of genetic counselors: a multinational survey. Am J Hum Genet 42:592–600.

Wolff G, Jung C (1995) Nondirectiveness and genetic counseling. J Genet Counsel 4:3–25.

13

Notes and Reflections

As a child I had difficulty figuring out the various relationships in my extended family. It was never clear to me who belonged to whom and my parents, as caring as they might have been, were rather taciturn about the subject. Thus, to this day, I have never fully mastered my family tree and it is only with difficulty that I can figure out which particular relative should be placed on which limb of the family, to whom I am related by marriage and who not. All that confusion eventually attracted me, as an undergraduate, to the logic of genetics.

It was later, in the mid-1960s, as an assistant professor in the Department of Psychiatry at Stanford School of Medicine that I became involved in genetic counseling. I came to Stanford as a postdoctoral fellow fresh out of Columbia University, where I had received a Ph.D. as a *Drosophila* behavioral geneticist, one of Theodosius Dobzhansky's last students. My only familiarity with genetic counseling came from Curt Stern's text in human genetics and from a brief exposure to Franz Kallmann and his group at the Psychiatric Institute of Columbia-Presbyterian Hospital in New York.

My mental image of genetic counseling was unformed. I knew that geneticists sometimes were called upon to do it. I certainly had no sense back then that someday I would be devoting my life to this field.

By the mid-1960s human genetics had taken several major steps forward. Just a few years earlier Watson and Crick had elucidated the structure of DNA, and the genetics revolution was underway. In 1959, Lejeune had developed techniques to study human chromosomes and had shown that trisomy 21 was responsible for Down syndrome. It seems incredible to recall that shortly before Lejeune's work the widespread belief held by biologists was that the diploid number of human chromosomes was 48!

In the 1960s, it became apparent that by combining karyotyping and amniocentesis, an innovation that had also then recently been developed, it would be possible to harvest fetal cells and study their chromosomal makeup. This opened the way for the prenatal diagnosis of chromosomal disorders. Modern genetic counseling had been born.

Two pediatricians at Stanford, Drs. Howard Cann and Luigi Luzzati, teamed up with an obstetrician, Dr. Doug Goodin, to start a genetic counseling clinic. Howard, if memory serves me correctly, ran the laboratory where karyotyping was conducted. Doug did the amniocenteses. Also involved with the clinic was a social worker, Rose Grobstein, who played multiple roles, one of which was to provide advice, comfort, and support to both patients and professionals on a regular basis. I joined their staff as a volunteer counselor and later on the four of us were joined by Dr. Elizabeth Short, who had an appointment in the Department of Medicine.

I began my counseling career by sitting in as an observer in sessions conducted either by Luigi or Howard. Eventually I conducted genetic counseling sessions of my own under Rose's watchful eye and it wasn't too long before I realized I hadn't a clue as to what I was doing. It was clear to me that most clients were not understanding the details of chromosomal disorders, technical procedures, and risk figures in the way we geneticists wanted them to (or hoped they would). The party line of the time was, "If they only had more biology and courses in statistics they would understand the information we provided." The genetic counseling literature back then was replete with such statements. It was the customer-is-always-wrong approach. Nonetheless, clients seemed to hang onto everything I said, as if it was a matter of life and death. What they seemed to grasp at was any indication of reassurance, anything that might suggest they would have a healthy baby.

As medical centers became more aware of the liability risks they had in offering prenatal diagnosis and counseling, the chances of providing reassurance to clients lessened. We had (and still have) to tell them about all the things that possibly might go wrong in the procedure and in their child's chromosomal makeup. We tried to convince ourselves that it would be sufficiently resassuring to our clients if we reiterated the statistical fact that 98% of time everything would turn out all right. Delusional thinking on our part! But, I'm getting ahead of myself.

I remember the first time I had to give "bad news" to a couple whose fetus was detected as having a trisomy. The chromosomal results always came out on Fridays and our protocol required the counselor to call that day and convey the news to the couple. Most often we would tell them, "Hello, I've got good news for you. The chromosomes are normal." But, this time I had to say, "I'm sorry but we found some problem and we would like you to come in Monday morning and discuss it with us."

After making the call, I felt awful and as the weekend progressed I couldn't help but think how I had really loused up the couple's weekend, how "crazy" and uncaring our protocol was, and other depressing thoughts. Finally, the full impact of how much pain I had inflicted on the couple came home to me. I began to understand how poorly prepared I had been to deal with human suffering. Scientific training and knowing biological and statistical facts no longer seemed enough. That weekend made me aware that there was more to genetic counseling than science. It transcended science. It was all about being human. Genetic counseling, I learned, concerned the dark side of life and that our work as professionals was to help humans prepare for, and when it happened, deal with the darkness.

Monday morning came and Rose and I met with the couple. They looked as if they had already gone through hell. I was anxious and fumbled for the right words and, after I showed them the karyotype and explaining the findings, Rose, thankfully, took over the session. The couple cried and held each other and I sat stoically and silent. I think back at it now, some 25 or more years ago, with shame and regret about my aloofness and unresponsiveness. I gave them information, but not a grain of solace. Rose, on the other hand, reached across the table and took the woman's hand into her own and spoke words of comfort. It was not long afterwards that I enrolled in my first course on counseling principles and practices.

This was a turning point in my life. Frankly, it was difficult learning to think like a counselor rather than as a geneticist or researcher. I just wasn't very good at it. My knee-jerk response was to seek for solutions of problems—quick fixes rather than a deeper understanding of the other person's experience. It took many stumbles and mistakes to learn how to help someone find answers—assuming there were answers to find—to their problems, theirs not mine.

One of the basic things you learn as a counselor is to reflect back what you hear the client say. But that means you have to listen to them, not to the interior chatter going on in your own head. And reflecting back your understanding of what they said also meant understanding their feelings at the time, not just that they were feeling sad or confused, but the shade of sadness and confusion, its depth, its width and height, its volume. This is something I still struggle with and confront personally each time I work with a client. But in this ongoing struggle one learns when to keep one's mouth shut and when to speak and, most important, how to say the things the client may need to hear with respect and kindness.

In retrospect, I believe I learned less from course work than from watching Rose or other experienced clinicians work with clients. Early on it became clear to me that, with a few notable exceptions, medical geneticists were not good role models. Their counseling skills generally had the same deficiencies as mine and, frequently, they had even greater difficulty handling emotionally charged issues than I did. However, they had greater face-to-face experience with clients and so even if I didn't understand (or like) what they said, it was an opportunity to learn what and what not to do. It was a time in which we were all learning.

By the mid-1970s my eyes were set on a career shift into clinical psychology. I knew that I wanted to combine my previous training in genetics with my growing expertise in psychology. Although my path was not yet clear, it was obvious that genetic counseling was the arena in which the two naturally came together.

In 1975, I invited myself to a conference on genetic counseling held in Colorado Springs. The proceedings of the meeting eventually were published as *Genetic Counseling*, edited by Herb Lubs and Felix de la Cruz. It was there I met colleagues—Ray Antley, Jim Sorenson, Arthur Falek, and one or two others—who shared some of my concerns about the direction in which the field of genetic counseling was headed. The overwhelming majority of attendees at the conference were physicians, many of who believed in various combinations of directive approaches or had a strong antipathy toward what psychology had to offer. Most could not see anyone but a physician doing genetic counseling.

One of the things many participants realized at the conference was that there was going to be a vast increase in demand for genetic services and that the existing number of providers was woefully inadequate. It was not long afterward that a genetic counseling training program was started at Sarah Lawrence College and the era of the genetic associate was born. Similar training programs were started at the University of California at Berkeley and at Irvine, the University of Wisconsin, and at Rutgers University.

It was around this time that Clarke-Fraser published the definition of genetic counseling, which has become one of the most cited papers in the field. It was clearly a definition drawn up by a committee, which evidently incorporated many compromises. I had (and continue to have) misgivings about it. It is too long, too complex, and evades too many obvious things, especially the psychosocial nature of genetic counseling, which, although hinted at in the definition, is never truly addressed. To this day I do not understand what the phrase "a process of communication" means. Defining genetic counseling this way suggests that human beings are irrelevant to what goes on; it could be two machines communicating to one another about genetic risks. The human element, the relationship aspect, the interaction between human beings all seem eliminated. The word "human" appears later in the definition as a euphemism for psychosocial and its placement in the definition suggests that it was a very subordinate activity relative to the communication of diagnostic and risk information. In my mind, the definition reflects a reluctance to touch, even in a tentative way, the affective nature of the actual work of genetic counseling.

In 1976, Pat St. Lawrence, the director of the Genetic Advising Option at the University of California at Berkeley, stepped down to return to her research and teaching in the Department of Genetics. At the time, the Option was located in an experimental unit, the Health and Medical Sciences Program, and genetic counseling was one of the curricular options. I applied unsuccessfully for the directorship. The job went to an academic psychologist with no experience in genetic services who proceeded to harangue the medical geneticists associated with the program with the "proper" way to conduct genetic counseling. Needless to say it was a fiasco and before the academic year was out, a search for a new director was carried out. This time I got the job.

I came to the directorship of the Berkeley Genetic Counseling Program—the first thing I did was to change its name—with a clear idea of how genetic counselors might be trained so as to emphasize their counseling role in genetic services. I insisted that each face-to-face encounter with genetic counselees be tape recorded so that there would be a realistic base on which the student's skills could be built. Initially there was some resistance to this practice and arguments were made that clients would never allow it, that doctors would never allow it, supervisors would never allow it, and so on. I had more patience then than I have now and so I stuck to my guns and argued back: "How do you know if you've never asked them or if you've never tried it? Try it. You may be surprised. They may be more willing than you think. You might actually come to like it."

The problems around tape recording were more in the mind than on the ground. Clients almost always gave permission to be taped so long as it was presented to them as a way of the student learning to be a better counselor and with the promise that the tape would only be heard by the student, the student's classmates, and supervisors. They almost always felt that they were making a contribution to the student's education and fostering the excellence of the field or were somehow being treated in a special way. It was also their way of giving something back, almost as a thank you, for the help they were receiving.

Slowly, supervisors came around. They understood that although a novel innovation in training (for genetic counselors), making tapes might actually help students learn counseling skills. Students were more threatened and hence more resistive. I knew that if my first class of students could be convinced, a precedent would be established. So I worked hard and eventually they too came around.

As expected, students were more self-conscious and so certain predictable patterns became apparent. The first tape or two presented for supervision generally were blank because the record button had not been activated. "I know I pushed the record button" was the ubiquitous excuse; I heard it from every student. The next pair of tapes were often inaudible or poorly recorded and the student had to learn that tape recorders are partial to the babbling of a squealing infant, or a background television set (if the recording was made in someone's home) rather than to adult voices. After a week or two, they got the hang of it and from then on it was smoother sailing.

Like most other genetic counseling programs, the Berkeley program had a 2-year curriculum. I taught the advanced genetic counseling seminar in the second year of the program. In the seminar, each student in turn would present a case and play a portion of their tape recording that they felt illustrated some particular issue or with which they had some difficulty. We would usually role-play such difficulties and discuss the personal and interpersonal dynamics involved. I would often point out the parallel processes of the clients and the student. Just as the student felt embarrassed in exposing their work to their supervisor or teacher, so too the client felt exposed in talking about their family history and relations. My thought was that if the student could come to master their feelings, they could not only understand their clients on a deeper level, they might also be able to help the latter feel less shame when dealing with genetic disease.

For some students, especially those who had relatives with some disability or genetic problem, the parallel processes were often painful. Invariably, we want to believe that we have worked through our past traumas only to discover, when faced with a situation that re-opens our wounds, that we still have more work to do. Someone who wants to be an effective professional in our field cannot hide from this psychological task without paying a price (e.g., personal limitation, the possibility of future upset, countertransferential inappropriateness).

My students would select one tape each semester and transcribe it verbatim from beginning to end along with process notes focusing on the possible psychological issues being discussed in its content. I'm sure they all hated doing it at the time, but years later several told me that the exercise had been a valuable part of their learning experience. It was an eye-opener to see on paper the actual words exchanged in the counseling session and to have an opportunity to contemplate how they might have done it differently if they had a second chance. And inevitably, with some other client, that chance arose.

In the back of my mind was the hope that my students would learn enough about the counseling profession to be outstanding professionals and would carry forward—in their work and in their own teaching—a philosophy of genetic counseling that emphasized its human aspect. I have always had the sense that what we do in genetic counseling has a near-religious purpose and that is to relieve, whenever possible, the sum of human suffering. Despite my many shortcomings, mistakes, misjudgments, and inadequacies—and as I grow older these all become more painfully apparent to me—I am sustained by the belief that I have succeeded, even if it has been in a limited way, in having an impact on a few students who, to my immense satisfaction, have gone on to surpass me.

After my retirement I found that I had more to say about genetic counseling and my vision of it. The years 1985 through 1990 were especially creative ones, a period in which I wrote some 12 papers, several book reviews, assorted letters to editors, and a book on the psychological aspects of coronary bypass surgery. I resumed my private practice in clinical psychology and continued to work with family members of patients with Huntington Disease (HD). In 1980 I volunteered to conduct a support group for the local chapter of the Huntington Disease Society of America and affected persons and their relatives made up about one-third of my practice.

In a sense, the Psychological Aspects of Genetic Counseling Series represents my eclectic interests both in research and clinical issues. The original two articles (Chapters 1 and 2) were an attempt to show how one might take a stab at qualitative and quantitative research on the process of genetic counseling. I had the naive idea that by publishing a real-life transcript of a genetic counseling session, the floodgates would open and others would willingly follow by sharing their work and experiences. The purpose of these articles was to break the seal on the black box, a tradition that long ago had already been established in every field of personal counseling and psychotherapy. Yet, here it is, nearly 20 years later and we have not moved forward very much in this regard. This is not a good sign. It suggests many possibilities—including a lack of self-confidence, an overblown fear of peer criticism, inadequacies of skill, and shame—none of which speak positively to the competence of professionals in the field.

The third article (Chapter 3) turned to the issues of guilt and shame in the genetic counseling context. The paper came out of class discussions with my students on the ubiquity of these responses among the clients they worked with. Much of the thinking on guilt and shame comes from the psychodynamic literature—often dense and filled with psychoanalytic assumptions and jargon—which is unlikely to be studied by genetic counselors. One student, Patricia Ward, attempted a term paper on the subject, a rather good one if memory serves me correctly, and with some of my own case material, my wife (also a clinical psychologist) and I put our heads together and came up with a draft in which we differentiated between the two psychological processes and attempted to show how to work with them in genetic counseling. The case material was still rather skimpy but when we gave it to Pat she added her thoughts and fleshed out the examples for the next draft. A little more editing and voila, Number III (Chapter 3)!

In the fifth paper (Chapter 5), I developed the idea of the preselected patient. It was an extension of the identified patient idea, which was prevalent in the family therapy literature, to the field of genetic counseling. I remember feeling fearful about submitting the article to a genetics journal because it seemed so "soft" in its conceptualization. But John Opitz, the editor of the *American Journal of Medical Genetics*, one of the truly great men in the field of medical genetics, encouraged me. He said that as soon as he read the article, it was as if a light of recognition went on in his mind. The paper was written over one weekend and went through minimum revision before I submitted it.

I had already begun to work on a review of the genetic counseling literature from a psychologist's viewpoint when Gerry Evers-Kiebooms' own review article appeared. Number VI (Chapter 9) merely fleshed out the literature subsequent to her excellent review.

I had the honor of being on the initial editorial board of the *Journal of Genetic Counseling* and wrote Number VII for the first issue, expressing my germinating thoughts on directiveness (Chapters 11). The problem of directiveness (D) and nondirectiveness (ND) continues to plague the field of genetic counseling. My first attempt to change the discourse on the topic was directed at focusing attention on D and ND as counseling strategies. My thought was to try to remove or tone down the moral aspect of the subject in which ND was invariably seen as Good and D as Evil. D is the legacy of an idea that professionals had near-omnipotent powers of persuasion. It was present in the eugenics movement. It was reflected in the traditional doctor–patient relationship. Few would disagree that it is culture-bound and weighted heavily with dubious moral values. My question is, "Does it work?" The evidence, pro or con, just isn't there. It probably does work under certain circumstances for some people, and in such instances it might be employed judicially. Does it work for everyone? Probably not. But, might not the same things be said for ND? ND, largely an American invention, is surely culture-bound and not suited for many parts of the world in which the professional advising role is strongly expected. Then again, what does ND mean? Is it only the absence of D? How is a professional to know when D is absent? These were some of the issues I had begun to lose sleep over in the early 1990s. Writing was a way to achieve sleep; hopefully the same is not true for the reader.

Essay VIII on suffering and countertransference (Chapter 4) came out of a talk I gave at a meeting of West Coast genetic counselors. It represents a first attempt to bring together some ideas about the nature of the blocks the professional brings with him or her to the expression of empathy. The thesis is hardly original: suffering is an inevitable part of being alive and until we suffer some combination of defeat, humiliation, and loss, we are not fully human. Nor can we understand the suffering of others.

Beginning with IX (Chapter 10), and elaborated further in X, XII, and XIII (Chapters 6, 7, and 8), I attempted to present a comprehensive case for a genetic counseling based on psychological principles and methods, and, through case examples, tried to help working professionals acquire more sophisticated counseling skills. The arguments against using psychological approaches in genetic counseling often boil down to the statement, "There just isn't enough time." This is a specious argument because, even if it could be demonstrated empirically that the statement were true—and it is important to note that there is no such evidence—more skillful counseling would be a time-saver and not a waste of time as some might have us believe.

I do believe that genetic counseling has to be made more effective with greater attention to the time investment involved. Better skills invariably save time and effort and provide more effective help to counselees.

The time argument is part of the mythology of genetic counseling. Essay XI (Chapter 12) deals with another myth, that regarding the impossibility of nondirectiveness. It is based on a talk given at an annual meeting of genetic counselors held in San Francisco in 1996 and was dedicated to the memory of Beverly Rollnick, an early leader in the field. In this paper I attempt to redefine the issues involved in directiveness and nondirectiveness in a way that liberates counselors to make the interventions they need to make in specific circumstances. One of the major thrusts of the paper is to separate advice-giving and directiveness and to demonstrate how advice might be rendered in a nondirective way.

I look back at my involvement in the field of genetic counseling with considerable satisfaction. Yet, self-doubt remains. Have I made an impact? Have I left a legacy? Perhaps I need to comfort myself with the belief that I have left something solid behind that will serve as building blocks for future developments. Future readers will decide whether or not I've made the best of the opportunity I had.

Index

Abortion
  counseling about. *See also* Directiveness
    transcript of, 8–9, 11–12, 14–15
  as issue in amniocentesis, 117
Accentuating the positive, as shame-
  alleviating tactic, 53
Advice, counselees' perception and use of,
  147, 153, 160
Advice-giving, 76. *See also* Directiveness
  nondirectiveness and, 153, 159–160, 161,
  172
Alliance, counselor–counselee. *See*
  Working alliance
Amniocentesis
  abortion as issue in, 117
  counseling before
    shame and, 42
    transcript of, analysis of, 1–18
  education-oriented counseling about,
    studies of, 116–117
Anencephaly, education-oriented counseling about, studies of, 117
Anger. *See also* Rage
  in shame reaction, 41
Anxiety, counselees', effect of genetic
  counseling on, 12, 20, 132
Approval, voicing, to counselees,
  75–76
Aspartylglucosaminuria, education-oriented
  counseling about, outcome studies
  of, 115–116

Associations, mental, in countertransference, 64
Attribution, in Bales system (for interaction
  process analysis), 21, 23, 23t
Attributional errors, counselees', management of, 42–43
Authority. *See also* Directiveness
  for absolution, as guilt-alleviating tactic,
    44, 45, 49
  in teaching model of genetic counseling,
    136
Autonomy
  counselees'
    nondirective counseling and, 153
    reinforcement of, 75
    teaching model of genetic counseling
    and, 136
  Erikson's concept of, 40
Avoidance, in shame reaction, 56

Bales system (for interaction process
  analysis)
  application to transcript analysis, 20–22,
    31–33
  application to transcript analysis
    (continued)
    category analysis in, 23–24
    content analysis in, 25–27, *26*
    sequence analysis in, 25, 25f
    strengths and limitations of, 32–33
  attribution in, 21, 23, 23t

Bales system *(continued)*
  categorization in, 20–21, 22t, 22–23
  cognitive-affective dimension in, 31
  scoring procedures in, 20–22
  task-oriented dimension in, 31
  unitization in, 20–21, 22, 22t
Behavior change
  genetic counselor as agent of, 17,
    99–100, 147–148
  persuasive coercion and, 151–152
Berkeley Genetic Counseling Program,
    168–169
Beta-thalassemia trait
  education-oriented counseling about
    outcome studies of, 116
    process studies of, 121–122
  family planning after counseling about,
    outcome studies of, 128
Boundary problems, 66

Categorization, in Bales system (for inter-
    action process analysis), 20–21, 22t,
    22–23
Clarification
  as advanced counseling technique, 76–78
  and advice-giving, comparison of, 76–77
  client's cognitive style and, 77
  client's language and, 77–78
Client-centered counseling, 82–83, 153
Coercion, in directiveness, 152–153
Comfort-giving, to counselee, by counselor,
    104–105
Communication, in professional–client rela-
    tionship, 85–86, 147
Compensation, and shame, 38
Competitiveness, in genetic counselor, 162
Confession, and relief of guilt/shame reac-
    tions, 43–44, 53
Consolation, of counselee, by counselor,
    104–105
Content-oriented counseling style
  indicators of, 27–28
  limitations of, 17–18
  operational definition of, 27
  quantitative analysis of, 20, 27–28, 31
Contrition, and relief of guilt/shame reac-
    tions, 43
Coping, in genetic counseling, 12
Counseling. *See also* Genetic counseling
  advanced techniques for, 73–83
  advice-giving and, 76
  clarifying procedures in, 76–78
  content-oriented. *See* Content-oriented
    counseling style

directive. *See* Directiveness
disclosure in, 66
education-oriented. *See* Education-
    oriented counseling
as focus of genetic counseling. *See*
    Counseling model, of genetic
    counseling
interview procedures for, 73–76
nondirective. *See* Nondirectiveness
praising and commending clients in, 75–76
prescriptive. *See* Directiveness
qualitative aspects of, operational mea-
    sures of, 20
reframing in, 78–81
role-playing in, 81–83
Counseling distance. *See* Working distance
Counseling interventions
  definition of, 36n
  for global (cosmic) guilt, 47–49, 58
  for guilt/shame reactions, 36, 44–53, 170
    case illustrations of, 43, 46–53, 54–61
    general methods for, 43–44
    preparation for, 43–44
  for iatrogenic guilt, interventions for,
    49–50
  for less advanced forms of shame,
    56–57
  for mixed shame and guilt, counseling in-
    terventions for, 43, 57–58, 58–61
  for more advanced forms of guilt,
    50–51
  for more advanced forms of shame,
    54–56
  for reduction of shame, 36
  for shame in couple, 56–57
  for unconscious guilt, 51–53
Counseling model, of genetic counseling,
    136–137
  arguments against, 107
  assumptions underlying, 136–137,
    137t
  counseling skills needed in, 139–140
  counseling tasks in, 137, 137t
  effects on professional, 139–140
  empathy and decency in, 99–107
  goals of, 136–137, 137t
  strengths and limitations of, 139–140
  and teaching model, comparison of,
    138, 138t
Counseling session
  clients' expectations for, ix–x
  content of, ix–x, 1
  control of, analysis of, 20, 30–31
  dynamics of, 1

specific intervention (transaction) serving as turning point in, quantitative analysis of, 20, 28–30, 29t, 32
structure of, 1
transcript of. *See* Transcript
warm-up period for, 12
Counseling skills
basic, x, 85–86, 155–156
in counseling model, 139–140
of genetic counselors, x–xi, 82
analyses of, from transcripts, 86–96, 169–170
flexibility needed in, 97, 144
inadequacies of, 85–86, 154n, 154–156, 161
in interview, 144
needed in future, effect of technology on, 96
nondirective, 161–163
in teaching model, 139–140
Counselor. *See* Genetic counselor
Counselor–counselee relationship, 11–18
directiveness and, 146
quantitative analysis of, 20, 28, 31–32
Countertransference, 97, 98, 171
associative, 64
management of, 67
professionals' experiences of, 63–64
projective, 64
sex selection and, 67
Couple
differences in concerns between husbands and wives in, 13
shame in, counseling interventions for, 56–57
Criticism, of genetic counselor, counselor's management of, 76

Decency, in genetic counseling, 101–102
Deception, in directiveness, 152–153
Decision making
effects of genetic counseling on, 19, 145, 147–148
facilitation of, clarifying procedures in, 76–78
use of information in, 111–112
Defenses
associated with guilt, 38–39
associated with shame, 38, 56
Denial, and shame, 38
Depression
counselees', effect of genetic counseling on, 20
in preselected individual, 70

Diagnostic issues, education-oriented counseling about, effectiveness of, 112–123
Directiveness, 151–153, 171
appropriate application of, 144
argument for, 144–146
coercion in, 152–153
counselees' expectations for, 144–145
and counselor–counselee relationship, 146
counselor's awareness of his or her strategy in, 144
covert, 143
deception in, 152–153
definition of, 143
effectiveness of, research on, 147–148
and empathy, 146
forms of, 152
goal of, 144
and interview, 144
limitations of, 86–89, 97
and nondirectiveness, comparison of, need for research on, 145–146, 171
and nondirectiveness, similarities in, 143
operational definition of, 142
as persuasive coercion, 152
phenocopies of, 152
research on, 147–148
sex differences in, 151
subtle, 143
Disclosure, in counseling, 66
Displacement, and shame, 38
Down syndrome
education-oriented counseling about
outcome studies of, 112–118
process studies of, 118–119
transcript of, 5–6, 11–12, 14–15
family planning after counseling about, outcome studies of, 124, 126
Duchenne muscular dystrophy, family planning after counseling about, outcome studies of, 125

Education-oriented counseling, ix–x, 82, 85, 135–136. *See also* Teaching model
disadvantages of, 14–15
and empowerment of counselee, 99
information transfer in, 111
limitations of, 17–18
literature on, review of, 111–123
outcome studies of, 112–118
process studies of, 118–123

Education-oriented counseling *(continued)*
 recall of information after, research on, 111
 recognition of information after, research
  on, 111
Educator, genetic counselor as, 16–17. *See
 also* Education-oriented counseling;
 Teaching model
Ego-bolstering, as shame-alleviating tactic,
 53
Ego ideal, 37
 shame and, 38, 58
Emotions, of counselees
 counseling tactics for dealing with,
  99–107
 genetic counselor's skill at dealing with,
  15–16, 93–96
 teaching model of genetic counseling
  and, 136
Empathy, 171
 directiveness and, 146
 effects of projective identification on, 65
 expression of, by counselor, 99–107
  need for, 12–13
 skillfulness needed in, 89–93, 97–98
Empowerment, of counselee, in genetic
 counseling, 99, 100–101

Facilitator, genetic counselor as, 17, 36. *See
 also* Directiveness;
 Nondirectiveness
Family coping strategy, in Huntington's disease, 68–72
Family dynamics, in Huntington's disease,
 71–72
Family planning, effect of genetic counseling on
 outcome studies of, 124–129
 process studies of, 129–132
 research on, pitfalls of, 123–124
Family system, and suicide in Huntington's
 disease, 71–72
Feelings, evoking, as shame-alleviating tactic, 53

Genetic counseling. *See also* Counseling
 agenda discrepancies for counselors and
  counselees in, 123, 147
 appraisal of, 19
  quantitative methods for, 33. *See also*
   Bales system (for interaction
   process analysis)
 central issues of, differences in counselors' and counselees' perception
  of, 123, 147

content variables of, 1–2, 15, 16
content versus process focus of, 16–18,
 99–100, 106–107
counseling model of. *See* Counseling
 model
definition of, ix
different styles of
 effectiveness of, research on, 116,
  120–122, 123
 outcome studies of, 116
 process studies of, 120–122
as educational process, x. *See also*
 Education-oriented counseling
effectiveness of, 109
 research on, 116, 120–122, 123,
  147–148
historical perspective on, 165–168
process variables of, 1–2, 15, 16
psychological approaches in, 73–108,
 135–140, 171–172
psychological process of, x, 1–18,
 99–107
psychotherapeutic considerations in, x–xi
session. *See* Counseling session
teaching model of. *See* Education-
 oriented counseling; Teaching
 model
time limitations and, 171–172
Genetic counseling literature. *See* Literature
Genetic counselor
 as agent of behavior change, 17, 99–100,
  147–148
 competitiveness in, 162
 counseling skills of. *See* Counseling
  skills
 criticism of, counselor's management of,
  76
 directiveness of, 16–17, 20, 171. *See also*
  Directiveness; Nondirectiveness
 quantitative analysis of, 20, 30–31, 32
 as educator, 16–17. *See also* Education-
  oriented counseling; Teaching
  model
 as facilitator, 17, 36. *See also*
  Directiveness; Nondirectiveness
 as information giver, 16–18
 and interventions for guilt/shame reactions, 36, 170
 as member of clinical team, 13, 15
 neutrality of, 16–17
  counselees' perception of, 147
  teaching model of genetic counseling
   and, 136
 passivity of, 83

special function of, 15
training of, 15–16, 66, 82–83, 96,
    139–140, 162–163
    content of, 169–170
    historical perspective on, 166–170
Guidance. *See* Directiveness
Guilt
    and affective reactions, 38
    in ambiguous situations, 43
    assessment of, 36, 43–44
    cognitive elements in, 44
    components of, 35
    in context of genetic counseling, 35,
        41–43, 170
    counseling interventions for, 36, 44–53,
        170
        case illustrations of, 43, 46–53, 54–61
        general methods for, 43–44
        preparation for, 43–44
    defenses associated with, 38–39
    developmental issues in, 39–41
        effects on guilt-alleviating tactics, 45
    duration of, 35, 43
    factors that evoke, 35, 43
    global (cosmic), counseling interventions
        for, 47–49, 58
    iatrogenic, 42
        counseling interventions for, 49–50
    less advanced forms of, 45
    more advanced forms of, 45
        counseling interventions for, 50–51
    prophylactic measures for, shortcomings
        of, 36
    realistic
        management of, 45
        versus unrealistic, 37
    and shame
        differentiation of, 37–38, 170
        mixed, counseling interventions for,
            43, 57–58, 58–61
    stages of moral thought and, 39–40
    unconscious, counseling interventions
        for, 51–53

Hemophilia, family planning after counsel-
    ing about, outcome studies of, 125,
    129
Hiding behavior, in shame reaction, 42, 56
Huntington's disease
    family coping strategy in, 68–72
    family dynamics in, 71–72
    informing children about, role-playing
        for, 81
    preselection in, 68–72, 170–171
    psychological changes seen in, presymp-
        tomatic family dynamics and,
        71–72
    suicide in, 71–72
        family system and, 71–72

Information
    recall of, after counseling, research on,
        111, 123
    recognition of, after counseling, research
        on, 111
    transfer of, in counseling, 111
    used in decision making, 111–112
        cognitive processes and, 123
        personal meaning and, 112
Information giver, genetic counselor as,
    16–18. *See also* Education-oriented
    counseling; Teaching model
Information-guidance genetic counseling.
    See Directiveness
Intellectualization, and guilt, 39
Interaction process analysis. *See* Bales
    system (for interaction process
    analysis)
Interview
    advanced techniques for, 73–76
    counseling skills needed in, 144
    directiveness and, 144
    history-taking style of, disadvantages of,
        13–14
Isolation, and guilt, 39

Learning-oriented counseling. *See*
    Education-oriented counseling;
    Teaching model
Limiting liability, as guilt-alleviating tactic,
    45
Literature
    on education
        outcome studies, 112–118
        process studies, 118–122
        review of, 111–123
    on reproduction
        outcome studies, 124–129
        process studies, 129–132
        review of, 123–132
    review of, 109–132, 171
        difficulties of, 110–111

Maternal age, education-oriented counsel-
    ing about, studies of, 116
Memory
    recall, 111
    recognition, 111

Mental retardation of unknown cause
  education-oriented counseling about, out-
    come studies of, 112
  family planning after counseling about,
    outcome studies of, 124
Message, implied, counselor's, transmitted
  to counselees, 17
Metamessage
  counselee's, addressing, 12–13, 32
  counselor's, transmitted to counselees,
    17, 88
Moral thought, stages of, 39
  correlation with measures of guilt,
    39–40

Narcissistic injury, and shame, 41, 57,
  58–61
Neural tube defects
  education-oriented counseling about,
    studies of, 117
  family planning after counseling about,
    outcome studies of, 129
Neutrality, of genetic counselor, 16–17
  counselees' perception of, 147
  teaching model of genetic counseling
    and, 136
Nondirectiveness. *See also* Rogerian counseling approach
  as active strategy, 160–161
  and advice-giving, 153, 159–160, 161,
    172
  appropriate application of, 91–93, 144,
    171, 172
  clarifying procedures used in, 77
  components of, 160–161
  counseling skills needed for, 161–164
  counselor's awareness of his or her strat-
    egy in, 144
  definition of, 143, 153
  and directiveness, similarities in, 143
  versus directiveness, need for research
    on, 145–146, 171
  examples of, 156–160
  goal of, 91, 143, 145
  historical perspective on, 150
  operational definition of, 142
  origin of, 153
  problems with, 154–156
  process of, 145
  research on, 147–148, 171
  sex differences in, 151
  trends in, 150–151
Normalization, as guilt-alleviating tactic,
  44, 45

Outcome research, 85
  on education, 112–118
  on genetic counseling, 1–2
    affective changes studied in, 19, 20
    information recall studied in, 19–20
    problems in, 20
    reproductive attitudes and/or behavior
      studied in, 19
    types of studies in, 19
  on reproduction, 124–129

Paradoxical interventions, use of, as shame-
  alleviating tactic, 54, 57
Patient preselection. *See* Preselection
Penance, and relief of guilt/shame reactions,
  44
Positive psychology, tactics of, in genetic
  counseling, 106–107
Positive reinforcement, of counselee,
  103–104, 161–162
Praise, of counselees, 75–76
Prescriptive counseling. *See* Directiveness
Preselection
  effects on preselected individual,
    70–71
  functions of, 70
  in Huntington's disease, 68–72,
    170–171
  mechanisms of, 69–70
  nonselected relatives and, 71
  phenomenon of, 68–69
Process research
  on education, 118–122
  on genetic counseling, 19
    need for, 20
    quantitative methods in, 33. *See also*
      Bales system (for interaction
      process analysis)
  need for, 107, 147
  on reproduction, 129–132
Projection, in countertransference, 64
Projective identification, in countertransference, 64–66
Psychotherapy, genetic counseling and,
  x–xi

Rage
  clients', management of, 66
  in shame reaction, 41, 56–57, 58–61
Rapport, establishing, in interview,
  73–75
Rationalization, and guilt, 39
Reaction formation, and shame, 38
Recurrence risk

clients' recall of, research on, 117–118, 122–123
family planning after counseling about, outcome studies of, 124–129, 131
Reframing
as advanced counseling technique, 78–81, 101
as guilt-alleviating tactic, 45, 80
in interpersonal conflict, 79–80
Repression, and guilt, 38
Reproductive intentions
agreement between spouses about, before and after counseling, research on, 130
certainty and uncertainty about effects on actual behavior, 127–128, 131
factors affecting, 127, 131
impact of genetic counseling on outcome studies of, 124–129
process studies of, 129–132
research on, pitfalls of, 123–124
literature on, review of, 123–132
risk perception and, 132
Research. *See also* Outcome research; Process research
on counseling skills, need for, 85
on directiveness, 147–148
on directiveness versus nondirectiveness, need for, 145–146, 171
on effectiveness of genetic counseling, 109–110, 147–148
on genetic counseling, methodological problems in, 109–110
on nondirectiveness, 147–148, 171
Responsibility, dual meaning of, 80
Risk
attitudes toward, effects of genetic counseling on, 19, 147–148
education-oriented counseling about effectiveness of, 112–123
outcome studies of, 114–118
information about, counselees' subjective experience of, 17
perception of
in genetic counseling, 147–148
and reproductive intentions, 132
recall of, studies on, 117–118, 122–123
subjective impression of, effects on reproductive planning, 130
Risky shift effect, 132
Rogerian counseling approach, 82–83, 153
Role-playing, as advanced counseling technique, 81–82

Self-directedness, counselees'
nondirective counseling and, 153, 161–162
reinforcement of, 75
Self-esteem
bolstering, in counselee, 161–162
techniques for, 99, 101–102, 103–104
lowered
in preselected individual, 70
and shame, 41, 57
regulation of, capacity for, 40
Sex selection, as countertransferential problem, 67
Shame
and affective reactions, 38, 44
anticipated, 42
assessment of, 36, 43–44
components of, 35
in context of genetic counseling, 35, 41–43, 170
counseling interventions for, 53–61
case illustrations of, 43, 54–61
general methods for, 43–44
preparation for, 43–44
in couple, counseling interventions for, 56–57
defenses associated with, 38
degrees of, 38
developmental issues and, 39–41
duration of, 35, 43
factors that evoke, 35, 43
and guilt
differentiation of, 37–38, 170
mixed, counseling interventions for, 43, 57–58, 58–61
less advanced forms of, counseling interventions for, 56–57
more advanced forms of, counseling interventions for, 54–56
ontogeny of, 40
reduction of, counseling interventions for, 36
self-system and, 38
Shame and doubt, Erikson's concept of, 40
Sickle cell trait, education-oriented counseling about, process studies of, 119–120
Silence, use of, in counseling, 95
Skepticism, counselees', effect of genetic counseling on, 20
Skills, counseling. *See* Counseling skills
Spina bifida, education-oriented counseling about, studies of, 117

Suffering, 171. *See also*
Countertransference; Empathy
Suicide, in Huntington's disease, 71–72
Superego, 37

Tape recording, of counseling sessions,
168–169
Teaching model, of genetic counseling,
135–136. *See also* Education-
oriented counseling
assumptions underlying, 135–136, 136t
and counseling model, comparison of,
138, 138t
counseling skills needed in, 139–140
effects on professional, 139–140
goal of, 135, 136t
limitations of, 139
psychological effects of teacher–student
relationship in, 136
Technology, effect on counseling skills
needed in future, 96
Thoughtfulness, in genetic counseling,
102–103
Time limitations, and genetic counseling,
171–172
Training, of genetic counselor, 15–16, 66,
82–83, 96, 139–140, 162–163

content of, 169–170
historical perspective on, 166–170
Transcript, of genetic counseling session,
analysis of, 1–18, 169–170
evaluation of counselor's skills in, 86–96,
169–170
process, 2
quantitative, 19–33
Transference, management of, 89–93,
97–98
Trust, in professional–client relationship,
146

Unitization, in Bales system (for interaction
process analysis), 20–21, 22, 22t

Videotapes, of genetic counseling, 1

Withdrawal, in shame reaction, 56
Working alliance, developing, as shame-
alleviating tactic, 53, 54, 57
Working distance, 83
definition of, 97n
development of, 97–98

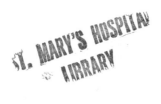